The World Health Organization was established in 1948 as a specialized agency of the United Nations serving as the directing and coordinating authority for international health matters and public health. One of WHO's constitutional functions is to provide objective and reliable information and advice in the field of human health, a responsibility that it fulfils in part through its extensive programme of publications.

The Organization seeks through its publications to support national health strategies and address the most pressing public health concerns of populations around the world. To respond to the needs of Member States at all levels of development, WHO publishes practical manuals, handbooks and training material for specific categories of health workers; internationally applicable guidelines and standards; reviews and analyses of health policies, programmes and research; and state-of-the-art consensus reports that offer technical advice and recommendations for decision-makers. These books are closely tied to the Organization's priority activities, encompassing disease prevention and control, the development of equitable health systems based on primary health care, and health promotion for individuals and communities. Progress towards better health for all also demands the global dissemination and exchange of information that draws on the knowledge and experience of all WHO's Member countries and the collaboration of world leaders in public health and the biomedical sciences.

To ensure the widest possible availability of authoritative information and guidance on health matters, WHO secures the broad international distribution of its publications and encourages their translation and adaptation. By helping to promote and protect health and prevent and control disease throughout the world, WHO's books contribute to achieving the Organization's principal objective – the attainment by all people of the highest possible level of health.

This publication is a contribution to the International Programme on Chemical Safety (IPCS). In addition, it is produced within the framework of the Inter-Organization Programme for the Sound Management of Chemicals (IOMC).

The IPCS, established in 1980, is a joint venture of the United Nations Environment Programme (UNEP), the International Labour Organisation (ILO), and the World Health Organization (WHO). The overall objectives of the IPCS are to establish the scientific basis for assessment of the risk to human health and the environment from exposure to chemicals, through international peer-review processes, as a prerequisite for the promotion of chemical safety, and to provide technical assistance in strengthening national capacities for the sound management of chemicals.

The IOMC was established in 1995 by UNEP, ILO, the Food and Agriculture Organization of the United Nations (FAO), WHO, the United Nations Industrial Development Organization (UNIDO), and the Organisation for Economic Co-operation and Development (OECD) (the Participating Organizations), following recommendations made by the 1992 United Nations Conference on Environment and Development to strengthen cooperation and increase coordination in the field of chemical safety. The purpose of the IOMC is to promote coordination of the policies and activities pursued by the Participating Organizations, jointly or separately, to achieve the sound management of chemicals in relation to human health and the environment.

IOMC

UNEP   ILO   FAO   WHO   UNIDO   OECD / OCDE

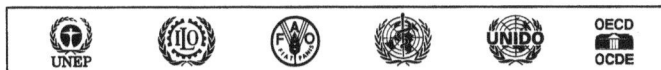

INTER-ORGANIZATION PROGRAMME FOR THE SOUND MANAGEMENT OF CHEMICALS

A cooperative agreement among **UNEP, ILO, FAO, WHO, UNIDO and OECD**

Guidelines for
poison
control

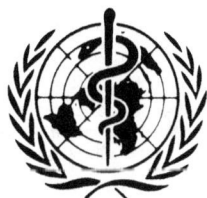

World Health Organization
Geneva
1997

WHO Library Cataloguing in Publication Data

Guidelines for poison control.

1. Poisoning — prevention & control   2. Poison control centers   3. Guidelines
ISBN 92 4 154487 2   (NLM Classification: QV 600)

Typeset in Hong Kong
Printed in Singapore
95/10529 — Best-set/SNP — 8000

Contents

Preface   v

Acknowledgements   ix

Introduction   xi

I. Policy overview

1. Poison information centres: their role in the prevention and management of poisoning   3

History   3

Functions   4

Benefits   10

Conclusions and recommendations   10

II. Technical guidance

2. Information services   19

Organization and operation   19

Location, facilities, and equipment   22

Staff   24

Financial aspects   27

Research   28

3. Clinical services   29

Introduction   29

Clinical toxicology units   31

Staff   33

Recommendations   36

4. Analytical toxicology and other laboratory services   38

Introduction   38

Functions of an analytical toxicology service   38

Location, facilities, and equipment   39

Staff   41

5. Toxicovigilance and prevention of poisoning   44

Introduction   44

Toxicovigilance and prevention programmes   45

Recommendations   47

6. Response to major emergencies involving chemicals   **50**

  Introduction   50

  Information   51

  Treatment   51

  Contingency planning   51

  Education and training   52

  Follow-up studies   52

  Financial support   52

  Collaboration between centres   53

7. Antidotes and their availability   **54**

  Introduction   54

  Scientific aspects   55

  Technical aspects   56

  Economic aspects   57

  Registration and administrative requirements   57

  Considerations of time and geography   58

  Special problems of developing countries   60

  Antidotes for veterinary use   60

  Improving availability   61

8. Model formats for collecting, storing, and reporting data   **64**

  Substance records   64

  Product records   64

  Communications records   64

  Annual reports   65

9. Library requirements for poison information centres   **66**

  Books   66

  Journals   71

  Publications of international organizations   72

  Computerized databases   73

  Educational material   73

Annexes

1. Summary description of the IPCS INTOX Package   77

2. Classified lists of antidotes and other agents   82

3. Example of a substance record: chemical   87

4. INTOX product record   91

5. INTOX communication record and miniform   95

6. Proposed format for a poison centre annual report   101

7. Environmental Health Criteria series   108

Preface

The International Programme on Chemical Safety (IPCS) was established in 1980 as a collaborative programme of the International Labour Organisation (ILO), the United Nations Environment Programme (UNEP), and the World Health Organization (WHO) in order to provide assessments of the risks to human health and the environment posed by chemicals, so that all countries throughout the world might develop their own chemical safety measures. The IPCS provides guidance on the use of such assessments and seeks to strengthen the capacity of each country to prevent and treat the harmful effects of chemicals and to manage emergencies involving chemicals. In its different activities, the IPCS collaborates with various international organizations and professional bodies. Its work on prevention and treatment of poisoning is undertaken in collaboration with the World Federation of Associations of Clinical Toxicology Centres and Poison Control Centres[1] and its member associations. The aims of the European Commission (EC) in the field of poison control are similar to those of the IPCS and many activities are undertaken jointly by the two bodies.

Poisoning by chemicals is a significant risk in all countries where substantial quantities and increasing numbers of chemicals are being used in the development process. Some countries already have well established facilities for the prevention and control of poisoning, many wish to establish or strengthen such facilities, and others have not yet fully recognized the extent of the risk.

The need for advice on poison control, particularly with a view to encouraging countries to establish poison information centres, was recognized at a joint meeting of the World Federation, the IPCS, and the EC, held at WHO headquarters, Geneva, from 6 to 9 October 1985. At this meeting it was recommended that guidelines be prepared on poison control and particularly on the role of poison information centres. It was also recommended *inter alia* that antidotes and other substances used in the treatment of poisoning should be evaluated, comparable information needed for diagnosis and treatment of poisoning collected and recorded in a standardized manner, toxicovigilance and poison prevention programmes developed, mechanisms for exchanging experience of dealing with major chemical accidents established, and specialized training in poison control encouraged.

A consultation of experts from poison information centres, from developed and developing countries, was held in London, England, from 24 to 25 February 1986, to advise on the structure and content of the proposed guidelines on poison control. It was agreed that the guidelines would be in two parts, the first concerned with national policy, and the second with technical aspects of establishing and running the various elements of a poison control programme. A drafting group was established and charged with the preparation of the guidelines. This group met twice — from 25 to 26 November 1986 in Brussels, Belgium, and from 16 to 20 February 1987 in London, England — and concentrated on the drafting of the policy overview.

---

[1] Hereafter referred to simply as the World Federation.

The initial draft was examined by an extended editorial group, meeting from 9 to 14 November 1987 in Salvador, Bahia, Brazil, during the Fifth Congress of the Brazilian Society of Toxicology. Work on the drafting of Part II was also initiated at that time.

Additional contributions were made by a number of experts, acknowledged below. Besides the extensive experience of poison control published in the literature, the results of the following activities were used in assembling material: the Joint IPCS/EC/World Federation survey on poison control centres and related toxicological services;[1] the Joint IPCS/EC Project on Antidotes; the IPCS Poisons Information Package project — IPCS INTOX — being undertaken jointly with the Canadian Centre for Occupational Health and Safety (CCOHS) and the Centre de Toxicologie du Québec (CTQ), with financial assistance from the International Development and Research Centre of Canada (IDRC); the joint WHO (EURO)/IPCS/EC meetings held in Munich, 16 to 20 December 1985, on public health response to acute poisonings[2] and in Munster, 8 to 12 December 1986, on prevention of acute chemical poisonings;[3] and the IPCS seminar on training for poison control programmes in developing countries,[4] held in London in February 1987.

Subsequently, a complete draft text was circulated for comment to members of the World Federation and selected IPCS focal points in various countries. The text was examined at a joint IPCS/EC secretariat meeting with the General Assembly of the World Federation, held at WHO headquarters in Geneva, 31 October to 2 November 1988; it was the opinion of the meeting that the guidelines reflected experience in Europe and North America, but should be tested in a number of other regions of the world before being finalized and published.

The guidelines were first presented at the Joint IPCS/WHO/World Federation Workshop on Prevention and Management of Poisoning by Toxic Substances, held in Kuala Lumpur, Malaysia, 29 November to 2 December 1989, in which representatives from 27 countries took part. They were also presented and discussed at two regional IPCS workshops on development of poison control programmes, held in Montevideo, Uruguay, in March 1991 and February 1992, organized by the Centro de Información y Asesoriamiento Toxicológico and with partial financial support from the International Union of Toxicology (IUTOX). The guidelines were further used as the basis for national workshops on poison control held in Ciloto, Indonesia, in November 1992, Bangkok, Thailand, in November 1992, and New Delhi, India, in December 1992.

Due account having been taken of experience of their use in different parts of the world, the guidelines are now issued as a WHO publication to encourage their wide distribution and use throughout the world.

Attention is drawn to the report[5] of the United Nations Conference on Environment and Development (UNCED), held in Rio de Janeiro, Brazil, in June 1992, in Agenda 21, Chapter 19, of which all countries are called upon to promote the establishment and strengthening of poison control centres to ensure prompt and adequate diagnosis and treatment of poisoning, including networks of centres for chemical emergency response.

---

[1] Report of the survey of poison control centres and related toxicological services 1984–1986. *Journal de toxicologie clinique et expérimentale*, 1988, **8**(5):313–371.

[2] *Public health response to acute poisonings: poison control programmes: report on a joint working group, Munich, 16–20 December, 1985.* Copenhagen, World Health Organization Regional Office for Europe, 1986 (Environmental Health Series, No. 11).

[3] *Prevention of acute chemical poisonings: high-risk circumstances: report on a joint WHO/IPCS/CEC meeting.* Copenhagen, World Health Organization Regional Office for Europe, 1987 (Environmental Health Series, No. 28).

[4] *Report of IPCS Seminar on Training for Poison Control Programmes in Developing Countries.* Geneva, World Health Organization, 1987 (unpublished document ICS/87.33, available on request from Programme for the Promotion of Chemical Safety, World Health Organization, 1211 Geneva 27, Switzerland).

[5] Adopted by the United Nations General Assembly at its 47th Session in New York, in December 1992, Resolution GA47/719.

Following the recommendations of UNCED in relation to sound management of chemicals, an Intergovernmental Forum on Chemical Safety (IFCS) was established in April 1994. One of the priority activities recommended to all governments by IFCS is the establishment of poison centres with related clinical and analytical facilities and the promotion of harmonized systems for recording data in different countries. These guidelines provide policy and technical advice to those responsible for setting up poison centres and related facilities, and give recommended approaches for harmonized data recording among countries.

Acknowledgements

The following are the members of the drafting group and experts who prepared specific sections of these guidelines:

Dr B. Fahim, Director, Poison Control Centre, Ain Shams University, Cairo, Egypt

Dr R. Flanagan, Toxicology Laboratory, Medical Toxicology Unit, Guy's and St Thomas's Hospital Trust, London, England

Dr M. Govaerts, formerly Director, Belgian Poisons Centre, Brussels, Belgium

Dr J.A. Haines, IPCS Secretariat, World Health Organization, Geneva, Switzerland (Chairman of the drafting group)

Dr V. Murray, Honorary Consultant, Medical Toxicology Unit, Guy's and St Thomas's Hospital Trust, London, England (Rapporteur of the drafting group)

Dr H. Persson, Director, Swedish National Poisons Information Centre, Karolinska Hospital, Stockholm, Sweden

Dr J. Pronczuk de Garbino, IPCS Secretariat, World Health Organization, Geneva, Switzerland

Dr E. Wickstrom, Director, Poisons Information Centre, Oslo, Norway

Ms H. Wiseman, Medical Toxicology Unit, Guy's and St Thomas's Hospital Trust, London, England

The following experts took part in consultations and review working groups for the guidelines:

Dr A. Berlin, Secretariat, Directorate General V, European Commission, Luxembourg

Dr I.R. Edwards, Director, WHO Collaborating Centre for International Drug Monitoring, Uppsala, Sweden, formerly Director, National Toxicology Group, University of Otago, Dunedin, New Zealand

Dr N. Fernicola, Toxicology Consultant, Pan American Health Organization, Bogotá, Colombia

Dr E. Fournier, formerly Director, Toxicology Service, Fernand Widal Hospital, Paris, France

Dr J. Garbino, formerly Assistant, Intensive Care Unit, Hospital de Clínicas Dr Manuel Quintela, Montevideo, Uruguay

Dr A.N.P. van Heijst, formerly Director, Dutch Poisons Control Centre, Utrecht, Netherlands

Dr J. Indulski, formerly Director, Nofer's Institute of Occupational Medicine, Lodz, Poland

Dr A. Jaeger, Director, Poisons Centre, Strasbourg, France

Dr J.P. Lorent, Swiss Toxicological Information Centre, Zurich, Switzerland

Dr S. Magalini, Director, Poisons Centre, Rome, Italy

Dr F. Oehme, Veterinary College, University of Kansas, Manhattan, KS, USA, formerly President, World Federation of Associations of Clinical Toxicology Centres and Poison Control Centres

Dr M. Repetto, Director, National Toxicology Institute, Seville, Spain

Dr L. Roche, Lyon, France, formerly Secretary General, World Federation of Associations of Clinical Toxicology Centres and Poison Control Centres

Dr B. Rumack, formerly Director, Rocky Mountain Drug and Poisons Information Center, Denver, CO, USA

Dr N.N. Sabapathy, formerly Zeneca Agrochemicals, Hazelmere, England

Dr S. Shabeer Hussain, Director, National Poison Control Centre, Karachi, Pakistan

Dr W.A. Temple, Director, National Toxicology Group, University of Otago, Dunedin, New Zealand

Dr M. Thoman, Associate Editor, Veterinary and Human Toxicology, Des Moines, IA, USA

Dr M.T. van der Venne, Directorate General V, European Commission, Luxembourg

Dr C. Vigneaux, Anti-Poisons Centre, Lyon, France

Dr J. Vilska, Director, Poison Information Centre, Helsinki, Finland

Dr G. Volans, Director, Medical Toxicology Unit, Guy's and St Thomas's Hospital Trust, London, England

Dr R. Wennig, Director, National Health Laboratory, Luxembourg

Introduction

The massive expansion in the availability and use of chemicals, including pharmaceuticals, during the past few decades has led to increasing awareness — on the part not only of the medical profession but also of the public and various authorities — of the risks to human health posed by exposure to those chemicals. Moreover, each country has a variety of natural toxins to which its population may be exposed. Authorities need only to consult local hospital accident and emergency departments for confirmation that toxic risks exist in every country and, in many cases, are increasing.

Tens of thousands of man-made chemicals are currently in common use throughout the world, and between one and two thousand new chemicals appear on the market each year. In industrialized countries, there may be at least one million commercial products that are mixtures of chemicals, and the formulation of up to one-third of these may change every year. A similar situation exists in the rapidly industrializing developing countries. Even in the least developed regions, there is growing use of agrochemicals such as pesticides and fertilizers, of basic industrial chemicals, particularly in small-scale rural cottage industries, and of household and other commercial products, as well as pharmaceuticals.

Every individual is exposed to toxic chemicals, usually in minute, subtoxic doses, through environmental and food contamination. In some instances, people may be subjected to massive, or even fatal, exposure through a chemical disaster or in a single accidental or intentional poisoning. Between these two extremes there exists a wide range of intensity of exposure, which may result in various acute and chronic toxic effects. Such effects clearly lie in the public health domain, particularly in cases of chemical contamination of the environment that may result in exposure of an unsuspecting public. The situation is similar to, but subtler than, exposure to infectious diseases: although chemicals may be absorbed in small quantities, they do not induce pathological signs until toxic concentrations are reached in the tissues of exposed individuals.

The global incidence of poisoning is not known. It may be speculated that up to half a million people die each year as a result of various kinds of poisoning, including poisoning by natural toxins. WHO conservatively estimates that the incidence of pesticide poisoning, which is high in developing countries, has doubled during the past 10 years; however, the number of cases that occur each year throughout the world, and the severity of cases that are reported, are unknown. It was estimated in 1982 that, while developing countries accounted for only 15% of the worldwide use of pesticides, over 50% of cases of pesticide poisoning occurred in these countries and, being due mainly to misuse of the chemicals, were largely avoidable. The worldwide frequency of major incidents involving chemicals, i.e. incidents that could cause multiple deaths, has been rising during the past two decades. There is growing concern about the possible health consequences of chronic exposure to naturally occurring toxic substances and to man-made chemicals and waste. In addition, poisonings of domestic animals are a cause for concern in certain countries, because of their economic impact on animal husbandry.

The principal toxic risks that exist in any country may be readily identified by surveys of hospital accident and emergency wards, forensic departments, and rural hospitals in agricultural areas. The growing incidence of poisoning from accidental exposures to chemicals, and recent examples of acute poisoning in local populations as a result of industrial and transport accidents involving chemicals have highlighted the importance of countries having special programmes for poison control and, in particular, the facilities for diagnosis, treatment, and prevention of poisoning.

Although the risks of poisoning by chemicals are not yet universally recognized, some countries have already established poison control programmes that provide the framework for both prevention and management of poisoning. These newly emerging programmes are important elements of chemical safety. Such programmes will vary in their structure according to local circumstances, but they all need clear direction and coordination in order to ensure the efficient use of resources, appropriate patient care, and effective preventive measures. There is a wide variety of starting points for any country wishing to initiate a poison control programme, and it is essential to identify the existing capabilities and facilities on which a programme may be built. The main elements of such programmes are identification of the toxic hazards existing locally (in order to establish preventive measures), diagnosis of poisoning, and treatment of poisoned patients.

These guidelines are intended to help countries that wish to establish or strengthen facilities for the prevention and management of poisoning. They are concerned with the identification of relevant existing facilities, of needs, of potential resources (including human resources), and of other bodies whose collaboration is essential to the implementation of successful poison control. Based on the experience of established poison information centres throughout the world, the guidelines provide advice rather than a unique model, and should be adapted in accordance with the socioeconomic and cultural conditions prevailing in each country.

Part I is written primarily for the administrator and decision-maker; it provides a policy overview of the problems of poisoning and the types of programmes and facilities that will be effective in preventing and dealing with them. Particular emphasis is given to the key role to be played by poison information centres.

Part II provides technical guidance for those with direct responsibility for the establishment and operation of specific poison control facilities and covers the following topics:

- information services
- clinical services (including lists of antidotes and other agents used in the treatment of poisoning)
- analytical toxicology services
- toxicovigilance and prevention of poisoning
- response to major emergencies involving chemicals
- antidotes and their availability
- standardized formats for the collection and storage of essential data by poison information centres
- documentary and library support for poison information centres.

I.

Policy overview

1.

Poison information centres: their role in the prevention and management of poisoning

History

Recognition of the problem of poisoning and of the need for specialized facilities to deal with it, as well as the existence of a number of health care professionals concerned with human toxicology, has invariably been the primary prerequisite for the establishment of poison information centres. The first centres were instituted in North America and Europe during the 1950s. Since then, numerous others have been created, principally in industrialized countries. The early poison information centres originated in a wide variety of fields, including paediatrics, intensive care, forensic medicine, occupational health, pharmacy, and pharmacology. To some extent, the original character of many centres has been maintained, and there is thus considerable heterogeneity in their structure and organization.

A global study undertaken during the period 1984–1986 indicated that, while most developed countries had well established facilities for poison control, this was rarely the case in developing countries.[1] Furthermore, in industrialized countries, there may be a number of institutions that provide different types of information on toxic chemicals. It must be remembered, however, that each ministry or agency in a developed country may have its own information services for its specialized needs, but that, in a developing country, the poison information centre — where it exists — may be the only source of information on toxic chemicals available 24 hours a day. Centres in developing countries may therefore have to provide a much broader toxicological information service than their counterparts in some developed countries.

Poisoning of animals may have important economic consequences, and special veterinary poison information centres have been established in some countries, including Australia, France, and the USA. In most countries, however, many poison information centres may deal with toxicological problems that affect both animals and humans.

Poison information centres may operate effectively with various types of organizational structure. The majority depend on a hospital administration and are, to some extent, connected with a university and with the country's public health service at national or regional level. Close association with units that treat poisoned patients and with analytical laboratories is essential to most centres, although the way in which this is organized depends on local conditions. Many centres are multifunctional, providing an information service, clinical unit, and analytical laboratory. Most are at least partially supported by public funding, and operate as independent foundations with their own governing bodies on which various public authorities are represented. It is thus impossible to specify a single organizational model for a poison information centre.

---

[1] Report of the survey of poison control centres and related toxicological services 1984–1986. *Journal de toxicologie clinique et expérimentale*, 1988, **8**(5):313–371.

Functions

The poison information centre is a specialized unit providing information on poisoning, in principle to the whole community. Its main functions are provision of toxicological information and advice, management of poisoning cases, provision of laboratory analytical services, toxicovigilance activities, research, and education and training in the prevention and treatment of poisoning. As part of its role in toxicovigilance, the centre advises on and is actively involved in the development, implementation, and evaluation of measures for the prevention of poisoning. In association with other responsible bodies, it also plays an important role in developing contingency plans for, and responding to, chemical disasters, in monitoring the adverse effects of drugs, and in handling problems of substance abuse. In fulfilling its role and functions, each centre needs to cooperate not only with similar organizations, but also with other institutions concerned with prevention of and response to poisoning.

Provision of information and advice

The main function of a poison information centre is to provide information and advice concerning the diagnosis, prognosis, treatment, and prevention of poisoning, as well as about the toxicity of chemicals and the risks they pose. As already mentioned, centres in some countries may be required to provide a very broad range of information on toxic chemicals, including data on risks to the environment and on safe levels in food and environmental media as well as in the workplace. The information should be available to all who may benefit from it, such as medical and other professional personnel, other concerned groups, various authorities, the media, and the public.

Access to the information service is normally by telephone, especially in an emergency, but there are several other communication channels, including computer networks, written responses to enquiries, and publications. Where telephone services are inadequate, the centre can act through direct consultation with those who visit in person and by providing written material on specific topics.

If it is to be reliable, the advice should be based on the continuous, systematic collection and evaluation of data by the staff of the centre, backed by local experience. All information and advice should be adapted to the specific circumstances of the suspected poisoning, i.e. whether exposure to the poison is acute or chronic, and the condition of the patient involved, taking into consideration the type of enquiry and the enquirer's technical understanding of the poisoning. While many routine enquiries may be answered by suitably trained nurses, pharmacists, or other specialists, supervision by a physician trained in medical toxicology is essential.

The information service must be available 24 hours a day, seven days a week, throughout the year. Section 2 provides further details of the role of centres in providing information.

Patient management

While a poison information centre may have its own clinical toxicology unit or treatment facilities, poisoned patients may be cared for at any of a variety of medical facilities: the centre will always provide information to a much larger area than that covered by a specific clinical toxicology unit. Many different categories of medical and paramedical personnel may be involved in the diagnosis and treatment of poisoning. Poisoning incidents frequently occur in the home, at work, or in rural areas and usually at some distance from medical facilities. The first person in contact with an individual who has been, or is suspected to be, poisoned may have little or no medical training.

Appropriate information has therefore to be made available to ensure an adequate response in every situation. It is necessary to confirm whether poisoning has actually occurred, to ensure that the proper first-aid measures can be taken, and to assess what type of treatment, if any, is required. The centre exists to provide such information, giving advice on the different aspects of diagnosis and treatment that is appropriate to the enquirer's level of understanding.

It is essential for poison information centres to be closely connected with facilities that provide care for poisoned patients and for the medical staff at each centre to be involved in the treatment of poisoning. This close association between poison information services and poison treatment services facilitates the necessary updating and expansion of information on the diagnosis and treatment of local poisoning cases, encourages detailed follow-up of patients, and stimulates essential research on human toxicology and patient management.

It is highly desirable that each country or major population area should have at least one clinical toxicology service dedicated exclusively to the management of poisoning cases and located in a hospital that can provide a wide range of services, including intensive care. Clinical toxicology services fulfil a specialized medical function in the management and treatment of poisoning, helping to improve the identification of toxins and evaluation of their effects, to elucidate the mechanisms and kinetics of different kinds of toxic action, and to assess new diagnostic and therapeutic techniques. They also play an important role in evaluating the clinical efficacy of antidotes. Clinical facilities are described in more detail in Section 3.

Rapid transport of severely poisoned persons to treatment facilities, or of doctors to patients who cannot be moved may be required. It is essential for poison information centres to be aware of the availability of ambulances — and possibly helicopters and aeroplanes — for transporting patients who need intensive care. Some ambulances and other means of transport may be specially equipped for transporting critically ill patients to the appropriate hospital facilities. In emergencies, coordination with the traffic police authorities may also be needed to help speed the transport of poisoned patients. Rapid delivery of antidotes and of samples for laboratory analysis must also be ensured, and could be coordinated by poison information centres.

Laboratory services

A laboratory service for toxicological analyses and biomedical investigations is essential for the diagnosis, assessment, and treatment of certain types of poisoning. It is especially important for clinical units treating poisoned patients: without analytical data, many toxicological problems cannot be accurately assessed. The data are required primarily to assist diagnosis and to back up decisions on the use of various therapeutic procedures to support prognosis. The laboratory service can also determine the kinetics of the toxin, particularly its absorption, distribution, metabolism, and elimination. Analytical facilities are also essential for research and for monitoring populations at risk from exposure to toxic chemicals. A laboratory service of the type outlined will permit the identification, characterization, and quantification of toxic substances in both biological and non-biological samples, i.e. in body fluids such as blood and urine, and in hair and nails, and in scene residues, as well as of both natural toxins and substances suspected of being poisonous.

If adequate general laboratory facilities already exist, it is possible to give general guidelines for the development of a service, although the requirements for particular analyses will vary with local circumstances. Two levels of operation may be envisaged. The first would offer a relatively restricted but more widely distributed service based mainly on simple spot tests, immunoassays, and thin-layer chromatography. Field tested techniques for use at this first level are detailed in an IPCS manual.[1] The second level would support the first but be more advanced, offering a full range of analyses using a wide variety of techniques. Laboratories operating at this level would be capable of acting as reference laboratories, confirming the results of screening tests and engaging in quality control and method development. Links should be developed between laboratories in such areas as training, research, and quality assurance.

The analyses to be developed should be selected according to proven clinical need and should:

- be backed up by a supply of appropriate pure reference compounds;

- be backed up by an adequate supply of consumables, such as reagents, and by satisfactory arrangements for maintenance; and

- use practical analytical techniques that can provide results within a reasonable time.

It may be economical and advisable for the laboratory to undertake other related work, such as the provision of services for monitoring therapeutic drug use, dealing with occupational chemical exposure, and screening for drug abuse, since these services require similar skills and can be undertaken with the same or similar equipment.

Adequate safety precautions must be taken to protect the laboratory staff from health risks, such as hepatitis and human immunodeficiency virus (HIV) infection, associated with handling biological samples.

A laboratory should have adequate staff and equipment to carry out the analyses that are essential in cases of poisoning within the country or region. Thus, an analytical toxicology service will need at least one trained analyst and one assistant, but larger numbers of personnel will be needed as the range of techniques in use and the number of analyses being performed increases. Analyses that are directly concerned with the treatment of poisoned patients should be available 24 hours a day.

Siting the laboratory in the same place as the poison information centre and treatment service has marked advantages as regards interdisciplinary collaboration. Many countries lack adequate toxicological laboratory facilities; in such cases it may be necessary to combine the services providing clinical analytical toxicology with those used in forensic medicine, occupational toxicology, monitoring of therapeutic drug use, food contaminants or substance abuse, and veterinary toxicology. Laboratory services are described in more detail in Section 4.

Teaching and training

The experience gained in a poison information centre can be an important source of human and animal toxicological data. The application and communication of this knowledge are vital for improving the prevention and management of poisoning. Centres thus have educational responsibilities that extend to the training of medical practitioners and other professional health workers likely to encounter cases of poisoning, and to communication with the local population and the mass media. Later sections of these guidelines include advice on the training needs of centres as well as on their teaching and training functions.

Toxicovigilance

Toxicovigilance is an essential function of poison information centres. It is the active process of identifying and evaluating the toxic risks existing in a community, and

---

[1] Flanagan RJ et al. *Basic analytical toxicology*. Geneva, World Health Organization, 1995.

evaluating the measures taken to reduce or eliminate them. Analysis of enquiries received by centres permits the identification of those circumstances, populations, and possible toxic agents most likely to be involved, as well as the detection of hidden dangers. The role of a centre in toxicovigilance is to alert the appropriate health and other authorities so that the necessary preventive and regulatory measures may be taken. For example, the centre may record a large number of cases of poisoning by a specific product newly introduced to the local market; cases occurring in a particular population group (e.g. analgesic poisoning in children); or cases occurring in particular circumstances (e.g. carbon monoxide poisoning from faulty heating stoves) or at particular times of the year (e.g. mushroom poisoning in the autumn or snake bites in the summer). Only now is the unique role of poison information centres in toxicovigilance being widely recognized. This role enables them to make a major contribution to the prevention of poisoning through their collaboration with the health and other appropriate authorities. Section 5 gives further details on this aspect of their work.

Prevention

Drawing on its observations and experience, a poison information centre can contribute to the prevention of poisoning by:

- alerting responsible authorities to circumstances where the risk of poisoning is high so that appropriate preventive measures may be taken, including: drawing the attention of various users of toxic chemicals to the risks involved, introducing codes of practice or legislation to control the labelling of toxic products or special packaging to reduce the risk of exposure to toxic substances, and modification or withdrawal of products from the market;

- encouraging manufacturers to employ less toxic formulations and to improve the packaging and labelling of their products;

- informing the general public, as well as special groups at risk, about recognized or emerging risks to the community posed by the use, transport, storage, and disposal of specific chemicals and natural toxins, and giving guidance on how to avoid exposure to, or accidents with, these substances; means such as brochures, leaflets, posters, educational programmes, and campaigns in the media may be employed, but should not arouse unjustified false anxieties and should take due account of local psychosocial and cultural circumstances;

- giving special warnings to professional health care workers concerning specific toxic risks.

The role of poison information centres in prevention of poisoning is described further in Section 5.

Drug information and pharmacovigilance

The medical profession must have access to advice on the therapeutic and adverse effects of pharmaceutical agents; some countries have drug information centres that provide this specialized information. Poison information centres are automatically concerned with problems of adverse drug reactions and side-effects, and may be contacted by physicians and the public for advice on both drug overdoses and the adverse effects of therapeutic doses. Enquiries may also relate to contraindications, for instance whether a drug should be prescribed in pregnancy or to a patient with a history of hepatic or renal disease. Poison information centres thus have the responsibility of contributing to pharmacovigilance in collaboration with other institutions established for that purpose. In a developing country, a combined drug and poison information service may be a logical use of resources.

Substances of abuse

All poison information centres receive enquiries about substances of abuse, including substances of natural origin such as cocaine, chemicals with a specific use such as solvents, pharmaceutical agents such as amfetamines, and illicit drugs designed for abuse. There are also increasing demands on analytical laboratories to identify substances of abuse. As many as 10% of patients seen at clinical toxicology facilities may be people poisoned by such substances; in some cases a mixture of substances may be involved, and in others the effects of one substance may be masked by those of another.

It is part of the task of a poison information centre to provide information relating to substances of abuse and, when necessary, to be able to refer enquiries or patients to institutions or authorities dealing with other aspects of substance abuse. Centres must know how to recognize the signs and symptoms of substance abuse, how to treat an overdose in an emergency, and how to deal with withdrawal syndromes. They must know what facilities are available for patients needing rehabilitation and for those who wish to give up substance abuse. Advice must be available for the families and friends of substance abusers on how to identify signs of intoxication and the substances involved.

Environmental toxicology

There is growing anxiety among the general public about the possible deleterious effects on health of toxic chemicals found in food, in consumer goods such as cosmetics, and in the environment (air, water, and soil). People are uncertain about whether pollution is giving rise to chronic poisoning among those exposed to it, whether the effects are cumulative, and whether there are long-term sequelae. Furthermore, the harmful effects on non-human species, and whether they may be acute or chronic, are of growing concern to both the scientific community and the public. Poison information centres, particularly in countries where there is no other readily accessible source of information on toxic chemicals, are being asked to provide information on the effects of environmental contaminants, on the risks associated with toxic wastes, and on safe levels of chemicals in the environment and in food and other consumer goods.

Poison information centres could play an important role in quantifying the relationship between exposure to toxic chemicals and observed clinical features of poisoning, including long-term sequelae. They should work closely with the medical profession, particularly general practitioners and occupational health physicians, hospital outpatient departments and pre- and postnatal clinics, who may be well placed to observe the possible clinical features and sequelae of exposure to chemicals. Medical practitioners must also be provided with data on the possible effects of exposure to environmental contaminants, and information on the types of biological and other samples that should be collected and analysed. Mechanisms for the systematic collection, validation, and follow-up of data should be established; it is also essential that the data are comparable, both nationally and internationally, so that they may be used for the benefit of all.

Contingency planning for chemical incidents and disasters

Poison information centres can contribute to the handling of major chemical incidents and disasters by providing appropriate information in the event of an emergency and by taking an active part in contingency planning and in education and training. They should also take part in epidemiological follow-up studies and other research initiatives, where appropriate, collaborating and acting in concert with other bodies involved in accident prevention and control. A national or regional poison information centre can serve to centralize and coordinate such activities. The role of centres in responding to chemical incidents and disasters is further described in Section 6.

Cooperation and interrelationships

To provide an effective information service and help in the prevention and management of the deleterious effects of toxic chemicals on human health and the environment, it is essential for centres to cooperate closely with a wide range of partners, particularly medical experts. Relationships should be fostered with other professional and social institutions that can contribute to the effective provision of information by poison information centres. For example, specialists in fields such as botany and zoology can assist in the rapid identification of toxic plants or animal species. Cooperation must also be established with industrial and commercial enterprises that manufacture, import, or handle chemicals, various research institutions, and consumer organizations and trade unions.

Contacts are needed with ministries of health and the full range of health services and institutions, including different hospital departments, general practitioners, paediatricians, pharmacists, coroners and medico-legal experts, occupational physicians, epidemiologists, experts in information technology, scientific societies, and local and central health authorities. It is also important for poison information centres to cooperate with other government bodies, such as ministries of agriculture, the environment, labour, industry, trade, and transport, and with consumer protection agencies.

Good relationships with newspapers, radio, and television are valuable, since the media have a key role in bringing information to the public. The publishing or broadcasting of educational messages on the prevention of poisoning can form part of a general process of health education; poison information centres should provide the media with appropriate information and material. In the event of a major chemical incident the media have an even more significant part to play: they must be kept fully and properly briefed by poison information centres and the emergency services so that all essential information can be given to the public without causing undue panic and alarm. In either role, the media have a responsibility to check the accuracy of the information they disseminate, so that any tendency to speculate or exaggerate is avoided. Regular contact between the media and poison information centres will lay the foundation for mutual confidence in the relationships.

Of equal importance is contact between the poison information centres themselves, both nationally and internationally. This may be established directly or through national and regional scientific and professional associations, as well as through the World Federation. Other means of contact include national and international congresses and meetings. Important areas for international collaboration are: exchange of case data and product and substance data in comparable formats, evaluation of antidotes, quality control, training, response to major accidents, and research.

Benefits

The service provided by poison information centres offers considerable direct health benefits by reducing morbidity and mortality from poisoning and enabling the community to make significant savings in health care costs. Cases of exposure to chemicals that carry no toxic risk can be rapidly identified, and unnecessary medical care and transport are thus avoided. Mild poisoning cases that can be treated by first-aid measures alone or by non-hospital medical personnel are quickly recognized, and physicians can be provided with advice on the management of moderately severe cases that can be treated in general health facilities. Severe poisoning cases, which may need very special facilities and equipment for treatment, are sent directly to hospitals where these facilities are available, thus avoiding delays and wastage of resources at general treatment facilities. Specific antidotes, therapeutic agents, and medical equipment can be made more easily available through coordination of stocks, so reducing costs and saving lives. Centres can also help to prevent the unnecessary use of special antidotes and of sophisticated and expensive treatments.

Access to information and advice at poison information centres stimulates the interest of local communities and makes them more committed to the prevention of poisoning. Centres help promote awareness of special requirements concerning the control and regulation of chemicals, including the labelling and packaging of products. Through active observation and evaluation of toxic risks and phenomena in the community, they are in a position to recognize sudden, unexpected rises in the incidence of poisoning and to alert authorities capable of taking the necessary action. Particular occupational settings may be involved, as well as the community in general. Indirectly, through improved prevention, the cost of poisoning to the whole community is reduced. Advice provided by centres in the event of major chemical disasters will help to minimize the effects on human health, maximize the effective use of limited medical resources, and prevent a recurrence of similar accidents. The education and training provided by poison information centres enable professional health workers and the general public to recognize and avoid the dangers of poisoning and to take effective action when poisoning incidents occur.

The case data collected by centres provide an epidemiological basis for local toxicovigilance and contribute to the international fund of knowledge about human toxicology and management of poisoned patients. Through its contacts with centres in other countries and regions, a poison information centre may obtain information, notably on antidotes, that has already been evaluated, thus enabling it to respond to emergencies and other needs in a cost-effective manner. It may also identify toxic risks evaluated elsewhere, so that timely preventive action may be taken.

Conclusions and recommendations

In accordance with WHO's definition of health and its goal of "Health for All by the Year 2000", everyone should have access to relevant information on how to prevent and deal with poisoning. Poison information centres provide such information and are an essential part of a country's capacity for ensuring the safety of chemical substances. Moreover, the United Nations, through its Conference on Environment and Development, has called upon all countries to promote the establishment of poison information centres with related chemical and analytical facilities to ensure prompt and adequate diagnosis and treatment of poisoning, including networks of centres for chemical emergency response.

Establishing a poison information centre

A poison information service should be available in *every country*, irrespective of its size or population. Ideally, there should be one national centre with, if necessary, a series of regional satellite centres. In a large country, or one with a large population or several different language groups, a number of regional centres may be needed, with close collaboration between them. Generally speaking, a poison information centre should serve a population of 5–10 million, but a proliferation of centres should be avoided. Depending on the availability of other services that provide information on toxic chemicals, a poison information centre may have to advise on a wide range of problems, and its associated facilities, e.g. laboratory services, may have to be multifunctional.

Location

When a poison information centre is established, especially in a developing country, existing medical facilities should be surveyed to determine where the centre can best be located and operate most effectively, bearing in mind that it is essential for a centre to have a number of health care professionals interested in human toxicology. Where feasible, the centre should be located at a leading hospital with emergency and intensive care services, as well as a medical library and a laboratory. If possible it should be linked directly with a hospital department where poisoned patients are treated: this may make it easier to recruit staff who already have experience and interest in the problems of poisoning. The laboratory facilities of such a hospital·can usually be expanded to allow toxicological analysis to be undertaken and appropriate quality control to be exercised. Location at a university teaching hospital or in a toxicological or public health institution may also have advantages. Whatever the location chosen, it should be the aim of the facility to operate 24 hours a day all year round.

Potential for development

A poison information centre needs certain minimum facilities and resources to function optimally, but a modest establishment that can be expanded in the future is preferable to no service at all. Initially, it may be impossible for the centre's own staff to provide a round-the-clock service, and arrangements may have to be made for an existing service, such as a hospital emergency ward, to help out at certain times. The aim, however, should be to provide a 24-hours-a-day, 7-days-a-week information service throughout the year, with continuous access to a physician trained in toxicology, and to achieve this as quickly as possible. The treatment and laboratory facilities at a hospital may be further developed to deal with poisoning cases. The information section of the centre should work closely with the clinicians and laboratory specialists but should remain an independent unit since it will serve a much larger community than the hospital — possibly the whole country.

Staff

A poison information centre needs a multidisciplinary team of poison information specialists,[1] led by physicians with toxicological experience. The team may include

---

[1] The term "poison information specialist" is used in these guidelines to include all personnel at poison information centres who are involved in providing the poison information service.

physicians, nurses, analysts, pharmacists, veterinarians, and other scientists representing a wide variety of disciplines including biology, chemistry, medicine, and pharmacology. This team needs the support of documentalists and such experts in information science and informatics as the circumstances and functions of the centre may warrant. A poison information specialist helps to prepare and provide expert information and advice on preventing and dealing with poisoning. While the scientific or technical background of this specialist may vary, the work demands appropriate training, which in some countries carries a certificate or other qualification. A poison information specialist should work under the supervision of a medical toxicologist. Those members of the team who answer enquiries must have adequate knowledge of toxicology and related scientific disciplines and should also be in regular contact with analytical and treatment facilities. The medical members of the team should themselves treat poisoned patients.

Medical personnel from emergency, intensive care, and treatment units may work part-time in the information unit, thus adding to their experience. There is growing recognition of the need for centres to have access to expert psychiatric advice, which is especially helpful in dealing with attempted suicide, the psychopathic use of poisons, and substance abuse, and in the management of some poisoned patients. Psychiatry may also provide guidance on dealing with emergency situations without causing panic, e.g. in the event of a major chemical disaster.

Good administration is of course essential. In some established centres, an administrative director is responsible for all administrative matters including funding, which allows the medical director to concentrate on the scientific supervision of the centre. Some form of administrative assistance is required at all centres, as well as adequate secretarial support.

Numbers of staff in the various categories must be sufficient to provide an adequate, continuous service at all times. While the enquiry load may vary according to the time of day, it would be desirable always to have a minimum of two poison information specialists on duty to answer calls. To provide continuous medical advice throughout the year, at least three trained physicians are needed.

Since highly experienced staff are essential, independent official recognition of the professional status of poison centre staff is desirable. Pay, working conditions, and incentives must be sufficiently attractive to keep staff turnover to a minimum. Further advice on staff requirements is provided in Section 2.

Equipment and facilities

If a poison information centre is to function effectively, certain basic equipment is essential, including suitable office furniture and facilities for the storage of confidential data. Specific areas should be set aside for answering telephone enquiries, consultation with patients, preparation of documents, staff meetings, and secretarial and administrative work. Staff on duty should have comfortable, suitably furnished rest areas. Additional desk space is needed at centres using computer equipment and on-line databases, and air-conditioning and humidity control may also be necessary. Centres themselves should be secure.

Equipment and facilities for the information service are described in detail in Section 2; equipment for treatment units is described in Section 3 and equipment for laboratory services in Section 4.

Poison information centres should have their own libraries and facilities for handling and reproducing documents. Reserved telephone lines are essential, and other means of national and international communication are highly desirable, such as telex, short-wave radio, and — in particular — fax. A fax machine is a recognized means of communicating information rapidly among centres and hospitals, particularly during emergencies, and should therefore be regarded as essential. Growing use is now being made of electronic mail for communication among poison control centres and other partners in poison control.

A list of handbooks and journals that are more or less essential for the information unit of a centre is given in Section 9, although each centre should add to and adapt this list in developing its own documentation and ensure that it is updated periodically.

Legal status and financing

Poison information centres should be officially recognized by government authorities. They should have independent status, stability, and neutrality to enable them to carry out their functions effectively. A centre may have a governing body, including representatives of various government and other authorities, to provide policy guidance and assist in fund-raising. This body should not, however, interfere with the daily operation of a centre or compromise its independence. The legal status of a centre should enable it to maintain the confidentiality of the data it handles. Its main source of financial support, which is a government responsibility, should respect its independent and neutral status. Information should be provided free of charge to enquirers, particularly in emergencies, although charges may be levied in certain circumstances.

Twinning arrangements

Twinning arrangements between centres in developing and developed countries can be very valuable, permitting exchanges of documentation, including case data on unusual types of poisoning, exchanges of staff for teaching and training, and the provision of antidotes, especially in emergencies. As a means of technical cooperation between developing countries, twinning should also be encouraged between new and established centres in these countries. For effective twinning it is important that centres have facilities for rapid communication (telephone, telex, and fax), and that arrangements are made to enable the rapid importation of antidotes and other essential supplies in times of emergency, without bureaucratic hindrance.

Action by national and local authorities

The prevention and control of poisoning could be made more effective through a number of appropriate actions by national and local authorities, where these have not yet been taken. These measures include:

- official recognition by government authorities of the role of poison information centres in carrying out toxicovigilance and of their contribution to prevention through the provision of information services, together with adequate financial support for the centres providing these services;

- ensuring that the community has ready access to the services provided by poison information centres;

- establishment of channels of communication providing prompt access for poison information centres to organizations (including the media) that can be alerted, outside normal working hours if necessary, to toxic hazards and advised on appropriate ways of dealing with them;

- ensuring that centres have access to adequate information on the composition of commercial and other products on the local market, on the understanding that the confidentiality of the information will be respected;

- ensuring that the information on patients gathered by a poison information centre remains confidential at all times;

- establishment of clinical toxicology services wherever needed;

- establishment of services for toxicological analysis wherever needed;

- provision of educational facilities and courses in toxicology, and establishment of certificates or other appropriate qualifications for information specialists at poison information centres, as well as for nursing and paramedical staff working in treatment units and analysts in toxicological laboratories;

- official recognition of medical toxicology as a discipline in its own right, and encouragement of academic institutions to develop the discipline by providing appropriate teaching units or departments;

- promotion of national and international exchanges of staff and experts;

- facilitating the exchange of biological and other samples for analysis, and the import and export of equipment and chemical reagents;

- provision of antidotes and essential supplies for the treatment of poisoned patients, and arrangements for their rapid importation in the event of an emergency;

- provision of transport facilities for patients where existing facilities are inadequate;

- improvement of the communications infrastructure in countries where it is inadequate; and

- establishment of mechanisms and facilities for the systematic recording and long-term follow-up of patients exposed to toxic chemicals.

Action at the international level

Cooperation at the international level between poison information centres, their national and regional associations, relevant professional bodies, governments, and international organizations in the following areas could do much to improve the prevention and control of poisoning:

- improving international communication and exchange of information and experience in the field of poison control, as well as exchange of personnel, particularly for purposes of education and training;

- harmonizing definitions of and criteria for clinical signs, symptoms, and sequelae of poisoning, including severity grading;

- establishing comparability between methods of collecting, storing, transporting, and analysing biological and other samples, and monitoring exposure to toxic chemicals and relating these to observed features of toxicity and sequelae;

- establishing internationally agreed mechanisms for the collection, validation, and analysis of data relating to exposure to toxic chemicals and observed features of poisoning, including long-term sequelae;

- undertaking collaborative research projects using agreed protocols, e.g. for evaluating new antidotes, elucidating the mechanisms of poisoning, and improving treatment regimens;

- establishing channels of communication between countries whereby antidotes, other therapeutic agents, and medical equipment can be made rapidly available on request in the event of a chemical incident or emergency, and samples for analysis can be imported and exported as necessary;

- establishing channels of communication between countries for rapid access to information about chemical incidents or emergencies that may be of value in deciding whether a toxic alert should be called.

II.
Technical guidance

2.

Information services

Organization and operation

The roles and functions of a poison information centre are briefly described in Section 1 of these guidelines. This section aims to provide more detailed guidance, principally on the establishment and operation of new centres, but also on the improvement of existing centres. It is additionally concerned with the location, facilities, and equipment of such centres and their staffing. Certain financial aspects are also considered.

The effective functioning of a poison information centre depends on the availability of an adequate volume of evaluated data to furnish a basis for the advice given. Two categories of data are collected: those derived from various external sources, including other centres, as well as scientific journals, textbooks, reports, and data sheets; and those obtained in the course of the centre's information work and its follow-up of reported poisoning cases.

It is essential for centres to have data on local commercial products, including pharmaceuticals, as well as on natural toxins produced by local poisonous plants and poisonous and venomous animals. Centres may be expected to identify tablets, capsules, plants, fungi, and insects and other animals. Each centre uses data culled from the various sources in compiling its own documentation for use by the staff of the centre. This documentation enables staff to provide information that is appropriate for the particular enquirer and adapted to local and national conditions. It is thus unique to the centre and essential for the information service that the centre provides.

Centres should establish a mechanism for obtaining access to adequate data on commercial products from manufacturers and importers; such data should be regularly updated and its confidentiality protected. A system of rapid access to data on foreign products is also essential. Information on the composition, packaging, and form of each product must be available and sufficiently detailed to allow the product to be identified, its toxicity evaluated, and its long-term effects assessed.

The documentation prepared by the centre itself on aspects of poisoning by chemicals and products, including evaluation of toxicity, symptoms, and treatment, is of particular importance. Past experience of poisoning cases involving specific chemicals and products plays an important role in this. Data on clinical cases, covering circumstances of poisoning, relevant medical histories, and the full evolution of each case, should be included in this documentation. Data on enquiries to the centre, as well as clinical data, should be systematically collected: they provide unique toxicological information that can be extremely valuable in diagnosis and treatment. To be of maximum value, case data must be fully recorded and followed up. Exchanges of such data between poison information centres, both nationally and internationally, could greatly enhance the effectiveness of the services they provide. A standard format for reporting case data and a mechanism for their collection and analysis are essential (see Annex 5).

Centres should also collect (and regularly update) information on health and other relevant resources and facilities in the region or country. This information should cover services that provide diagnosis and treatment, including specialized treatment facilities, such as dialysis units, hyperbaric oxygen chambers, and clinical toxicology services; analytical facilities and the types of analyses they provide; facilities for emergency transport of patients; antidotes and their availability; and other medical and non-medical services with related areas of responsibility.

A poison information centre should have its own library, which could be associated with a university or medical library. Certain books and publications should be accessible at all times at the centre itself; others could be kept at a local medical library but must be immediately accessible. Section 9 lists a selection of the books and journals that may provide library support for a poison information centre.

Poison information centres would benefit greatly from more efficient collection, storage, retrieval, and analysis of the data they require. Computerization is one tool for this purpose, and most established centres have their own computers. The IPCS has developed a computerized information package, known as IPCS INTOX, to help centres in developing their own poison information systems. A summary description of the package is given in Annex 1.

Planning a poison information centre

Identification of the principal toxic risks in the local community helps in determining the activities on which the efforts of a poison information centre should initially be concentrated (e.g. poisoning by pesticides). Available facilities should be reviewed to allow the selection of locations that best meet the criteria outlined in these guidelines. However, it must be stressed that primary prerequisites for the success of a centre are enthusiasm and interest in human toxicology on the part of a group of health care professionals who recognize the problem of poisoning in their country and are committed to dealing with it.

During the planning of a poison information centre, the following questions should be carefully considered:

- To whom will the service be offered initially, e.g. the medical profession only, the public, veterinarians? Will it be a 24-hours-a-day service from the outset? How will it be expanded subsequently? How will its existence be advertised to the user population?

- What are the initial and subsequent staffing requirements? How will the centre contact and recruit the necessary expertise?

- Are the telephone and other communication systems adequate?

- How will the centre collect the full range of data needed to operate the information service?

- How will the reliability, accuracy, and usefulness of the data be evaluated?

- How will the data be compiled, recorded, and stored for rapid retrieval?

- How will the data be managed and updated? Who will have access to what type of data, and who will have the authority to modify data files?

Before a centre becomes operational it is also necessary to:

- obtain certain essential literature (see Section 9);

- provide basic training for the staff who will work in the centre (see page 24);

- print forms (in the local language) for collecting information on local commercial products and for recording enquiries to the centre, with provision for follow-up of calls and cases (see Section 8); and

- on the basis of local information, begin compiling files on the chemicals used in local commercial products, including pharmaceuticals, on local natural toxins, and on relevant medical and analytical services available in the country (see below and Section 8).

Operating a poison information centre

Once a poison information centre becomes operational, i.e. is able to offer an emergency response service, it should function around the clock. In the initial period, before the centre is fully staffed, the service may, at certain times, rely on the assistance of established emergency or intensive care services.

For ethical and commercial reasons, much of the information handled by poison information centres, notably that relating to manufactured products and to patients, must be considered as confidential. Responsibility for the correct handling of such information rests essentially with the medical director and eventually with the other staff of the centre, particularly the information specialists who need the information on an emergency basis.

Rapid identification of the poisons or types of poison involved in an emergency is one of a centre's main tasks. The constitution, origin, uses, and toxicity of the pharmaceuticals, chemicals, plants, or animals involved need to be identified immediately to permit the appropriate action to be taken.

Information on commercial products

Most existing poison information centres began by organizing card indexes of basic information on each of the toxic substances or natural toxins used or occurring in the area or country concerned. Although this type of information can now be stored in rapidly accessible computer files, the use of card indexes may still be recommended in a newly established centre for the initial identification of poisons. A computerized system can be added later, and the card index system should therefore contain as much information as is needed, recorded in such a way that it can later be transferred to a computerized system. The recommended format for collecting and storing information on commercial products for use in the IPCS INTOX Package is given in Annex 4.

The card index or computer file should contain entries on *all* commercial products, such as pharmaceuticals, household products, and pesticides, commonly used in the country concerned. Although files from other (e.g. neighbouring) countries may be useful, every poison information centre will have to organize and maintain its own files. Information for these may be extracted from local pharmacopoeias and government registries, or obtained from pharmaceutical firms, manufacturers of household products, importers of chemicals, etc.

A similar card index or computerized file system should be organized for natural toxins, poisonous plants, and poisonous and venomous animals.

Information on enquiries

Systematically collected data on enquiries form an essential part of the database at a centre. They must cover not merely the enquiries that pertain to clinical cases but every kind of enquiry received at the centre, including toxicological consultations registered by the clinical services.

Standardized recording of enquiries, including those relating to clinical cases, will allow the centre to:

- maintain its own clinical and other data registry
- implement toxicovigilance activities
- support epidemiological and statistical studies
- perform self-audit and continuously evaluate the quality and efficiency of its services
- back up its clinical and legal responsibilities
- validate new techniques of patient management
- provide data for scientific reports
- exchange information with other poison information centres
- contribute to the fund of knowledge on human toxicology.

Computer facilities for recording data on enquiries and cases offer enormous advantages, and the IPCS INTOX package provides a framework for this purpose. Further work is needed on, *inter alia*, the classification of agents involved in poisoning, the standardization of analytical data, and the harmonization of severity grading of case data; much is being done at present by IPCS in collaboration with poison centres and experienced toxicologists. The format used in the IPCS INTOX Package for recording communications is given in Annex 5.

All poison information centres should prepare annual reports of their activities; a suggested layout for an annual report for a poison information centre is given in Annex 6. This layout provides a comprehensive format, which should be adapted to local circumstances.

Location, facilities, and equipment

Location

General criteria for the location of a poison information centre are given in Section 1 of these guidelines (page 11), but the final choice of location will depend on local circumstances. Certain conditions, however, should be respected, namely that:

- the centre is regarded as neutral and independent, and security for all the information stored at the centre is ensured;

- there is rapid and ready communication with other organizations concerned with poisoning, particularly clinical and analytical services;

- access to the centre within the building in which it is located is easy, but restricted for unauthorized persons; and

- the centre is centrally situated within the geographical and demographic area it serves.

The poison information centre should ideally be located within, or closely associated with, a hospital. Location within a hospital has the advantage of providing ready access to a network of medical disciplines that will support and enhance the work of the centre, enabling staff to deepen their knowledge of the clinical aspects of poisoning. If also located within a university, the centre will have easier access to, among other things, libraries, research facilities, and educational activities. Location within a public health institute or ministry permits more activities relating to prevention of poisoning and a closer relationship with decision-making authorities, but it is still essential for the medical staff of a centre to be involved in the care of poisoned patients, and for the information service to operate round the clock.

To some extent, the location may also be determined by the number of enquiries received. For example, if more than 5000 emergencies are registered each year, a full-time staff will be required to provide a 24-hours-a-day service, and the centre should then be an independent facility, though preferably situated in a hospital. However, some centres are run effectively from other locations. If fewer than 5000 calls are received annually, outside support may be required to maintain a 24-hour service. In this case also, the centre may be located in a hospital but should be situated where regular hospital staff, notably from emergency and intensive care wards, are available to assist in maintaining the service.

Facilities

A poison information centre should be accommodated in suitable rooms or working areas, equipped with basic furniture (desks, tables, chairs) and such other facilities as are essential for its principal functions. Additionally it should have immediate access to the relevant literature and other sources of information.

The rooms should be large enough to permit the efficient storage and retrieval of documents and the holding of necessary meetings. One room should be allocated to the "answering" service and should contain the telephones assigned to it, plus the basic files, protocols, and books needed by the information specialists and physicians on duty. An area should be set aside as a library where scientific work can be undertaken. Another area is required for working groups and staff or other meetings; this should be at least large enough to allow the assembly of all the staff of the centre, together with a number of advisers or visitors.

Staff on duty should have a private area providing the basic facilities for personal hygiene and rest. Food and drink should also be available, as well as vehicle parking space outside the building.

The medical director should have an office or suitable private area for specific work, interviews, and consultations; similar facilities should be available to other staff receiving patients. A separate area should also be assigned for administrative and secretarial work. As a centre develops new functions, additional space may be required and the location should therefore allow for this future expansion. Experience has demonstrated that, as more information is gathered and new activities or responsibilities assumed, bigger working areas rapidly become necessary.

Furniture

The minimum furniture needed for a new centre consists of desks and chairs, a large work table, lockable filing cabinets, and bookshelves. As the service develops and the working area grows, further appropriate office and library furniture should be provided. When the service starts functioning on a round-the-clock basis, the medical toxicologists and information specialists on duty must have a private area with suitable furniture and an adequate degree of comfort. It may also be necessary to provide a bed for rest between duty periods. Optimally, there could be specially designed work stations incorporating computer terminals where appropriate.

Equipment

It is particularly important that a poison information centre should have equipment for fast and reliable communication, and for the storage and retrieval of information.

Communication with enquirers must be through reliable telephones reserved for the purpose and covering the whole area served by the centre. Two telephones are a minimum. In some countries the poison information centre is automatically connected with the emergency telephone services, and all calls concerned with toxicological emergencies are directed straight to the centre. The emergency number of the centre should be easy to remember and accessible from all telephones in the region served by the centre. In developing regions of the world, the radio telephone can be useful in reaching distant areas and remote populations. Other rapid methods of communication include the telex and, for documents, the fax, now considered a "must" at most centres. Electronic mailing systems (e-mail) are now being established at some centres. Fast and reliable communication will be valuable not only for the information service but also for the necessary contacts with other centres and access to international databanks. These systems must be well maintained and financially supported by the appropriate authorities or government ministry. The importance of worldwide communication networks for toxicology has been recognized: ideally, the centre should be equipped with the most practical advanced communication system appropriate to the country and to the centre's functions.

The storage of case records, files, and documentation requires, at the least, sufficient bookshelves and filing cabinets to permit systematic collection and easy retrieval. A lockable section should be available for confidential data.

With the development of the service, additional space, furniture, and storage facilities should be made available for the growing collection of books, published material, and files. If circumstances permit, automated systems may replace manual storage, retrieval, and processing systems, and computers must consequently be recognized as important items of equipment for a poison information centre. A microfiche system may also be a useful means of storing documentation.

A poison centre often has to stock antidotes and other substances used in the treatment of poisonings and therefore requires a refrigerator; a lockable cabinet for storing pharmaceutical agents should be provided.

From the outset, a centre should be adequately equipped with typewriters, a word processor with a good quality printer, and photocopying equipment or other suitable means of reproducing documents. The role of a centre in education and training may require it to have its own slide, overhead, and video projection equipment.

Staff

A poison information centre should be headed by a director experienced in toxicology and have sufficient personnel to perform the duties of the centre on a 24-hours-a-day, 7-days-a-week basis. The director is wholly responsible for the operation of the centre and should ideally be employed on a full-time basis. He or she should have personal leadership qualities, together with the ability to supervise other staff and maintain good relations with colleagues and other collaborators in the poison control programme. The director should also be able to promote research, raise funds, and undertake the further development of the information service. The medical functions of the centre must be the responsibility of a medical toxicologist. It may also be desirable to have an administrative director responsible for the financial, administrative, and other non-medical aspects of the centre. In addition, full-time — and possibly also part-time — medical toxicologists, poison information specialists, and administrative and support staff are required. Ultimately, centres also need advisers in various medical and non-medical fields, few of whom would normally be on the staff of the centre at the outset. The work of the centre may eventually call for the services of a number of full-time or part-time experts in particular fields such as psychiatry and veterinary medicine.

In Part I of these guidelines it was pointed out that a fully operational centre, providing a round-the-clock service and adequate medical advice, requires a minimum of three full-time medical toxicologists (or the part-time equivalent) and a sufficient number of poison information specialists to ensure at least one person being on duty at any given time. The frequency of enquiries is likely to vary during the course of the day, and it may be necessary to have additional staff on duty at certain times. In this respect, patterns vary throughout the world, and it is up to the individual centre to ensure that its service is adequate for local needs. In practice, at least 6–8 dedicated, trained, full-time poison information specialists are required: this allows for coverage of staff absences for illness, holidays, and professional training.

The medical toxicologist

Medical toxicology is the discipline concerned with the harmful effects of chemicals, including natural substances, on humans, although its scope is broader than simply the clinical aspects of the subject. A medical toxicologist is a qualified physician with several years' experience in the treatment of cases of poisoning and a grounding in such areas as emergency medicine, paediatrics, public health, internal medicine, intensive care, and forensic medicine. Clinical experience in occupational diseases and in diseases caused by pollutants and other chemicals of environmental origin is particularly relevant. Experience in clinical toxicology is essential, and experience in toxicological research is also valuable.

The medical toxicologist may provide expert advice to national decision-making bodies, and is often responsible for training at hospitals and medical faculties, and takes part in the multidisciplinary teaching of toxicology at university level. He or she must keep abreast of the latest developments in all areas of the discipline, including analytical and experimental toxicology.

In the specific field of information, the medical toxicologist must be able to organize and compile a comprehensive dossier on poisons and their effects, based on the available material and personal experience, to train junior toxicologists and the centre's information specialists in collecting and interpreting data, and to give appropriate information in response to enquiries.

It is particularly important for medical toxicologists to undertake the systematic collection and evaluation of clinical observations, as these constitute a major source of information for the poison information centre.

The medical director of a poison information centre should be the most experienced of its medical toxicologists and the best equipped to take responsibility for medical decisions, treatment protocols, and the promotion of research.

The poison information specialist

For the purpose of these guidelines, the personnel directly in charge of the round-the-clock response to enquiries are termed poison information specialists. They must be appropriately trained and able to carry out the basic functions of a poison centre, with the support of a medical toxicologist, preferably a clinician treating poison victims. They should be able to give information to all types of enquirer on the basis of duly evaluated data available at the centre and in accordance with agreed patient management protocols. In cases where information is not available at the centre, they should know how it may be obtained. They must also know when to consult a medical toxicologist or adviser in a special area and should be able to record details of enquiries, cases, or consultations, using a standardized method. In many situations, poison information specialists will help evaluate the data used at the centre. With additional qualifications or experience in information management and computing, they can play a useful role in the organization and management of records kept at the centre.

Poison information specialists may be drawn from many different disciplines, including various branches of medicine, pharmacy, nursing, chemistry, biology, and veterinary science. In each case, training for the specialized work of a poison information centre is essential and should be a continuing process so that they all remain abreast of new developments in toxicology. Information specialists should have the opportunity to participate in appropriate scientific meetings in their own countries and elsewhere. Training should lead to an officially recognized certificate or other qualification: there is a need for universally recognized qualifications in this field.

All members of the information team should take part in the different activities of the centre, e.g. answering enquiries, preparing documentation and reports, operating computer programs, and making regular searches of the literature. Regular discussions among the team on interesting cases and various toxicological problems should be encouraged as a means of making each member aware of new developments and promoting a harmonized approach to poisoning and patient management. Periodic meetings among poison information centres within a country, or from the various countries of a region, should also be encouraged in order to discuss similar topics.

Veterinary expertise

The widespread use of veterinary drugs and the addition of chemicals to animal feedstuffs, unless carried out under veterinary supervision, can lead to contamination of human food. The effects of toxic substances on animals are often unique, and their diagnosis and appropriate management require the expertise of trained veterinarians. Furthermore, cases of exposure of animals to environmental chemicals may provide early warning of the potential exposure of humans. It would be highly desirable for poison information centres to have access to specialist veterinary knowledge in order to be able to recognize and respond to problems of animal poisoning as well as to advise on the risks of human exposure to drugs used for animals.

Administrative and support staff

A centre should have at least one secretary and, if possible, clerical staff to assist in the establishment, maintenance, and updating of the information system. Provision should be made for the maintenance and cleaning of equipment and facilities at the centre; this is often the responsibility of the administration of the building where the centre is located.

The administrative staff of a poison information centre should be qualified to manage and supervise its financial resources, equipment needs, and operational requirements, as well as dealing with routine personnel matters. Ideally, there should be a senior administrator or administrative director in charge of all these activities, with suitable support staff and clearly defined responsibilities that do not overlap with those of the medical director.

If a centre has its own library it will require a librarian or an information specialist/documentalist, or both.

Advisers in special areas

When a poison information centre is being established, a variety of specialist help and advice is essential. This may be medical or non-medical and may come from independent experts or from representatives of specialized organizations and local agencies. As the centre acquires more experience and the scope and volume of its work expand, it may become necessary to employ extra staff with some of the various kinds of expertise indicated below, on a part-time or full-time basis.

Specialists collaborating with the centre should be able to provide, whenever necessary, specific information on subjects within their recognized fields of expertise. The toxicology-related areas where the information might be needed will depend on local circumstances. Advice from the medical profession may be required in such areas as public health, psychiatry, occupational medicine, paediatrics, nephrology, teratology, anaesthesiology, veterinary medicine, pharmacy, epidemiology, and environmental health. Consultation with representatives of medical associations and government or local medical organizations may be of value whenever specific problems arise. In non-medical areas, advice might be needed from specialists in agronomy, botany, zoology, herpetology, entomology, mycology, ecology, statistics, computer sciences, industry, engineering, law, and information technology and other areas of information management.

A close relationship should be established, once those specialists able and willing to collaborate with the centre have been identified. An agreement should be made as to what is expected of the specialists, and how and when advice is to be provided to the centre. No special training is required for these collaborators, but they should be introduced to the work of the centre and the way it functions. Periodic joint scientific meetings and activities may be very helpful in cementing the relationships between the centre and its special advisers, who may also help in training the staff of the centre in their specific areas of competence.

Development of human resources

The evolution of the poison information centre will depend on local circumstances, needs, and resources. Ideally, there should be career opportunities for all the staff of a centre, each of whom should have the chance of additional training and advancement within his or her own area of competence. Contacts with other agencies dealing with various aspects of the prevention and treatment of poisoning should be stimulated both within the country and abroad. Where appropriate, professional staff should be encouraged to undertake relevant research and contribute to the literature.

Financial aspects

Since poison information centres can be considered as part of the public health service, government resources are the most appropriate source of financial support. However, each centre must remain neutral, independent, and preferably autonomous in order to carry out its functions effectively, and these conditions must be respected, whatever the principal source of financing.

Governments should recognize the cost-effectiveness of the service provided by poison information centres to the community, and therefore make every effort to sustain their financial support. It may be difficult for a centre to produce direct evidence of its cost-effectiveness, but it should be stressed that:

- it discourages the excessive use of medical resources
- it reduces the adverse effects of poisoning on health, as well as mortality from poisoning
- it helps to reduce the risks of occupational poisoning.

Other sources of funding may be acceptable, if they are available and if the autonomy of the centre is guaranteed. Social groups in the community, fund-raising campaigns, philanthropic groups, and associations of industry and commerce may all be sources of support. Funds for specific projects received from national and international organizations concerned with chemical safety may be very useful for investigating areas of joint interest. Private funding initiatives have proved to be effective in many countries and should not be discouraged, particularly in the case of new services.

It is an important principle that information should be provided free of charge, at least in an emergency. However, some payment to the centre may be appropriate when special reports or expertise are requested by private institutions or individuals.

Although the bulk of a centre's budget will be devoted to salaries, it should be remembered that adequate funding for the maintenance of up-to-date information is essential. Significant portions of the budget should also be devoted to the operation and maintenance of equipment, for example the telephones, telex, fax, photocopying, and computer systems, as well as to the development of appropriate educational material.

Research

Poison information centres are important sources of information on human toxicology; in particular, they may be able to signal the approach of new toxicological hazards. They also have enormous scope for broadening the scientific database on human toxicology through regional and international cooperation. Their research function should be recognized and encouraged by the relevant authorities.

3.
Clinical services

Introduction

Cases of poisoning may be treated in many places, e.g. at the scene of the accident, during transport, in a hospital. The type of care that can be given will depend on whoever makes the initial contact with the patient and in what circumstances. Certain members of the community, such as firemen, policemen, and teachers, may frequently be the first to be faced with poisoning cases. In rural areas, nurses and primary health care workers, and even agronomists and veterinarians, may have to deal with poisoned persons. They all need at least some basic training in first aid as well as in decontamination and measures for their own protection. An IPCS handbook on this first level of response to poisoning is in preparation.[1]

General practitioners or family doctors are often the first medically qualified persons consulted. They must be able to give appropriate initial treatment and may need to contact their local poison information centre. Most patients with serious poisoning, if they survive, will sooner or later reach a hospital, ideally one with a wide range of medical facilities, including intensive care. In some places, specialized treatment services have been established offering the best possible conditions for the management of poisoning. These services also have the advantage of ready access to a wide range of related medical facilities.

Most cases of poisoning, however, will be treated through a country's normal health service facilities, usually at a general hospital, far from a poison information centre and without access to a specialized clinical toxicology unit. According to patients' needs, treatment may be given by different services within the hospital, including the following:

- *Emergency services*. In practice, emergency services receive a relatively high number of poisoning cases, as they function on a round-the-clock basis and are provided with trained personnel and basic equipment for decontamination and life-support measures.

- *Intensive care units*. Intensive care units are usually well provided with highly specialized personnel and equipment for resuscitation, life-support measures, and care of critical poisoning cases.

- *General medical units*. Basic medical care of non-critical poisoning cases can be provided within general medical units in which staff have received some training in, or information on, clinical toxicology and which are in close contact with poison information centres.

- *Specialized services*. Specialized services offer the advantage of well trained medical staff and appropriate equipment for the management of poisoning cases in which

---

[1] *Management of poisoning. A handbook for health care workers.* Geneva, World Health Organization (in preparation).

specific organs or physiological functions are affected; they include nephrology, gastroenterology, neurology, cardiology, and haematology services.

- *Paediatric departments.* Poisoned children are frequently treated in paediatric departments.

To be able to treat poisoned patients, general hospitals need equipment for:

- gastrointestinal, cutaneous, and ocular decontamination (e.g. equipment for gastric lavage)

- immediate, and often longer-term, life-support measures (e.g. endotracheal intubation, assisted and controlled ventilation, parenteral fluid therapy, pharmacological treatment, cardiac pacing, defibrillation)

- continuous cardiac and circulatory monitoring (through ECGs, blood pressure measurements, etc.) and monitoring of other vital functions

- X-ray examinations

- initial and repeated general biomedical laboratory analyses (e.g. acid–base balance, blood gases, electrolytes, blood glucose, liver and kidney function, and coagulation)

- initial and repeated specific toxicological analyses of body fluids such as blood, urine, and stomach contents (the choice of analyses will vary according to local patterns of poisoning)

- haemodialysis, peritoneal dialysis, haemoperfusion

- administration of appropriate antidotes (some of which may be specific to local needs and all of which should be stored in accordance with WHO recommendations[1]).

In an emergency, it is essential that the relevant medical personnel at general hospitals and other health service facilities where poisoning cases are treated have rapid access to toxicological information and experience. Here, the poison information centre plays a key role through its telephone advice service. Ideally, centres should circulate information to general hospitals and other health service facilities on a regular basis. This information should be adapted to suit local needs and should include general advice on the diagnosis and management of poisoning cases commonly expected to be treated at the particular hospital or facility, as well as information on new developments in patient management and on new types of poisoning.

The information flow should be a two-way process. General hospitals and health science facilities should be encouraged to maintain close contact with national and regional poison information centres and to furnish these centres with regular reports on cases of poisoning, particularly the more unusual ones. Such reporting helps to maintain an up-to-date national database on poisoning and is important for toxicovigilance.

The training of medical personnel in relevant aspects of toxicology for their work in managing poisoned patients is another important task for the poison information centre. For this purpose, it is essential that the centre itself is closely involved in the management of poisoning cases.

Some countries have found it valuable to have one or more specialized clinical toxicology units where the most important cases of poisoning in a region are treated. In

---

[1] *The International Pharmacopoeia, Third edition. Vol. 2, Quality specifications.* Geneva, World Health Organization, 1981.

some cases an intensive care unit is associated with, or forms part of, a clinical toxicology unit. The latter would normally be associated with a national or regional poison information centre.

Clinical toxicology units

Roles and functions

While general clinical wards and various specialized services that treat both poison victims and other types of patient are potential participants in poison control programmes, clinical toxicology units deal exclusively with the management of poisoning. These independent specialized units may have three principal functions besides patient management, namely toxicovigilance, education, and research. Locating a poison information service and analytical facilities in the same department or building as a clinical toxicology unit is an advantage and may be of benefit to patients. However, where there is no common location, highly reliable communications between the unit, the information service, and the laboratory are essential in order to establish a partnership between them in the diagnosis and management of poisoning.

Ideally, a specialized clinical toxicology unit should be part of national or regional medical facilities for the management and treatment of poisoning. It provides for:

- optimal treatment of poisoned patients
- identification of the effects of chemicals and natural toxins on health
- evaluation of the cause–effect relationship in a case of poisoning
- assessment of new developments in clinical and analytical methods of diagnosis and in treatment
- development of specific therapeutic management
- appropriate follow-up and surveillance of cases for identification and assessment of sequelae, and
- study of the circumstances of the poisoning and predisposing factors (data can then be used for planning preventive action).

Clinical toxicology units should record data on poisoning cases and toxicological consultations in a standardized format, preferably compatible with that used by poison information centres (see Annex 5). Full case data, including follow-up, should be recorded.

Location and facilities

The minimum requirements for setting up a clinical unit for the treatment of acute poisoning are:[1]

- availability of methods, equipment, and areas for the resuscitation, decontamination, and initial management of poisoning cases
- good communication links with a poison information centre
- well established protocols for the treatment of common cases of acute poisoning
- availability of antidotes for immediate use, in quantities appropriate to the frequency of the main forms of poisoning (see Section 7)
- laboratory facilities for standard biological analyses and for toxicological screening (see Section 4)

---

[1] See also Table 1, page 32.

- availability of emergency transport for patients
- an emergency plan for dealing with disasters and major chemical accidents.

To function to the best advantage, a clinical toxicology service should be located as a separate department within an advanced multifunctional hospital and within or next to the poison information centre, preferably on the ground floor in order to facilitate rapid access. It should have:

- full facilities for prolonged life support, stabilization of vital signs, and correction of acid–base and fluid and electrolyte abnormalities (see Table 1)
- equipment for decontamination and the elimination of poisons, including dialysis and haemoperfusion

Table 1
Facilities for clinical toxicology

	Minimal facilities	Optimal facilities
Location	Emergency department; internal medicine ward; or intensive care unit with ready access to a poison information centre	Separate specialized unit within a multifunctional poison centre, or closely associated with such a centre with two-way links
Equipment for: Resuscitation	Devices for: suction; airway control; and IV administrations	Additionally: mechanical ventilator; ECG; oscilloscope; defibrillator; pacemakers; haemodynamic monitoring equipment
Decontamination	Separate area for decontamination, with gastric lavage equipment, shower, and facilities for skin and eye washing	Additionally: facilities for dialysis and haemoperfusion
Diagnosis and prognosis		EEG; fibroscopic devices, e.g. oesophagoscope, bronchoscope
Antidotes and other agents	Selection made from the list in Annex 2, according to local needs	Full selection, including agents still under development
Laboratory: Biological	Blood typing; cross-matching; blood gases; pH; electrolytes; standard uring analysis; cerebrospinal fluid analysis	Comprehensive analysis of blood, urine, and other body fluids; functional studies
Toxicological	Screening test equipment for thin-layer chromatography	Equipment for more specific quantitative and qualitative analyses, including those for toxicokinetic and various research studies (see Section 4)
Other facilities	Normal facilities for transport of patients	Transport facilities (e.g. ambulances, aircraft) equipped with life-saving systems Access to a specialized centre, e.g. for psychiatric and social rehabilitation
Personnel	Emergency room physicians and intensive care physicians, available 24 hours a day	Clinical toxicologists; anaesthetist; paediatrician; psychiatrist; social worker

- the appropriate range of antidotes and medicaments used in the treatment of poisoning (see Section 7)
- protocols for the assessment and management of poisoning cases
- access to an analytical laboratory with appropriate equipment for qualitative and quantitative biological and toxicological assays on a round-the-clock basis (see Section 4)
- protocols for recommended analytical tests, including collection of specimens and interpretation of results (see Section 4)
- established systems for the collection and analysis of data on all clinical cases for epidemiological records, toxicovigilance assessment, and preventive action
- psychiatric rehabilitation and social assistance services.

There should be sufficient space for all levels of patient care, and for the activities of the staff on duty, including administration, small conferences, education activities, and storage of clinical records.

Consideration should also be given to such practical matters as a comfortable rest area, personal hygiene facilities, parking space, and the provision of food and beverages round the clock for duty staff.

Staff

Initially, the staff may consist of emergency-room physicians to provide resuscitation and first aid, plus paediatricians, anaesthetists, and intensive-care staff to look after severely poisoned patients. However, in developing countries or in newly established clinical units, there may be a shortage of sufficiently well qualified medical personnel, in which case medical officers or adequately trained paramedical personnel have an important part to play in the initial evaluation, transfer, and referral of poisoning cases. They should be capable, for example, of recognizing a case of poisoning, of identifying the main toxic syndromes (e.g. anticholinergic, cholinergic, opioid), and especially of recognizing situations that require the immediate application of life-saving measures.

Ideally, therefore, the staff should consist of:

- The medical director of the clinical toxicology service, who should be qualified to:

  — organize the care of poisoned patients, both directly and through case consultation
  — implement, review, and update protocols for the evaluation and treatment of poisoning cases
  — supervise staff performance
  — promote toxicological research
  — identify those programmes or agencies that might provide funding for research or the further development of the service.

- Trained specialist(s) in clinical toxicology with practical experience and, ideally, with a professional qualification.

- Physician(s) with competence in the care of critically ill patients.

- Psychiatrist(s).

- Advisers from other medical disciplines, e.g. pharmacology, and from non-medical areas of interest.

- Social workers.

- Supporting paramedical staff (e.g. nurses, medical officers).

- Administrative staff and record-keepers.

Training

While the need for clinical toxicology services is becoming increasingly obvious, the growing demand for adequate, trained personnel is not being met. Physicians from countries with no appropriate facilities should be sent for training in toxicology to established centres where poisoned patients are treated. The objective in each case should be for the trainee to obtain experience of every aspect of the work of a centre, so as to be able to initiate or develop poison control activities in his or her own country. It is important for trainees to know the problems and special "risk profiles" associated with poisoning in their own countries before starting their courses.

Physicians from developing countries where facilities for training in some aspects of clinical toxicology are available could be trained in their own countries if appropriate programmes were organized, with visiting experts invited to teach those subjects for which training facilities are lacking. Alternatively, trainees could be sent to centres abroad to supplement or enlarge experience gained at home.

A training programme for clinical toxicologists should include education in the theoretical aspects of human toxicology, preparation for a dissertation, and teaching activities. Trainees should also gain experience of work in:

- a poison information centre (including training in preparing documents, collecting information, replying to enquiries, recording case data, and follow-up of cases);

- a clinical toxicology unit, emergency department, or intensive care unit where poisoned patients are treated; and

- a toxicological laboratory, where a practical understanding of sampling and analytical methods and of the medical interpretation of the results of analyses is provided.

There should also be opportunities to attend or participate in seminars, courses, lectures, conferences, and meetings within and outside the centre.

This training programme would be expected to take two years and should be undertaken preferably by physicians with some experience in related disciplines and some knowledge of chemistry, biochemistry, statistics, epidemiology, pharmacology, and information technology. It should cover all the main areas of toxicology in general, while stressing those in which local cases or risks of poisoning are frequent or severe. The basic contents of such a training programme are indicated in Table 2.

Although the basic professional training of clinical staff is supplemented by experience obtained in the course of their work, the rapid development of toxicology makes continuing education and updating of knowledge a professional and ethical responsibility. Means of achieving this include the reading of scientific literature, participation in local, regional, and national seminars, meetings, and workshops, or attendance at training courses of several days' or weeks' duration. The continued updating of expertise can be stimulated by, for example, making participation in scientific meetings a condition of certification. In the USA, where professional certification is controlled by the American Board of Medical Toxicology, the American Board of Veterinary Toxicology, and the American Board of Toxicology, evidence of active interest in new developments is necessary in order to maintain expert status in toxicology. This system not only encourages continuing education but also contributes to career advancement by boosting professional status.

Table 2
Contents of training programme on clinical toxicology

Part 1

1. *General principles of medical toxicology*

- Type and circumstances of poisoning:
  - — type of poisoning (acute, subacute, chronic)
  - — deliberate (suicidal, criminal, dependence, abortion)
  - — accidental (at work, at home, environmental)
  - — poisoning epidemics
  - — groups at risk (children, the elderly, pregnant women, workers)

- Basic principles of toxicology:
  - — experimental data and evaluation
  - — toxicity testing
  - — routes of exposure
  - — toxicokinetics (metabolism)
  - — toxicodynamics (mechansims of toxic action)
  - — carcinogenesis
  - — teratogenesis
  - — genetic toxicology

- Clinical diagnosis:
  - — clinical aspects
  - — toxic syndromes, differential diagnosis
  - — role of analytical services

- General principles of treatment of poisoning:
  - — first aid and decontamination
  - — prevention of absorption
  - — enhancement of elimination
  - — symptomatic and supportive treatment
  - — antidotal therapy

- Organizations and groups with a role in poison control programmes:
  - — governmental and regulatory authorities
  - — poison control centres
  - — universities
  - — experimental toxicologists
  - — other research groups concerned with assessment of human toxicity

2. *Human toxicology of specific substances*

- Systematic study of the most common and important causes of, and substances involved in, human poisoning:
  - — medical products
  - — industrial products
  - — pesticides/agricultural products
  - — household products
  - — poisonous plants and fungi
  - — poisonous and venomous animals
  - — environmental pollutants
  - — food poisoning

- For each substance, the following should be considered:
  main use; physicochemical properties; kinetics; metabolism; mode of toxic action; toxicity data; laboratory data (toxic levels, etc.); pathology; symptomatology; diagnosis; treatment; carcinogenicity; teratogenicity; legal aspects; prevention; particular aspects of acute and chronic toxicity; long-term effects

Table 2 (*continued*)

Part II

- Human toxicology: an extended study, including coverage of less commonly encountered substances
- Prediction of toxicity
- Statistical and epidemiological programmes for evaluation of acute and chronic toxicity of specific substances
- Critical evaluation of literature sources
- Medico-legal aspects
- Research: an appreciation of the methods used in experimental toxicology, toxicovigilance, and epidemiology
- Different areas of toxicology: ecotoxicology, occupational toxicology, immunotoxicology, genotoxicity, forensic toxicology, etc.

Nurses and paramedical personnel working in clinical units where cases of poisoning are treated should also be given special training in toxicology. This is especially important in countries where qualified physicians are scarce or are overwhelmed by crowded emergency rooms and outpatient consultations.

Nurses, paramedical personnel, and clinical officers will need a concise and more practical training course than that given to physicians, perhaps based on the training programme on clinical toxicology outlined in Table 2. For example, the principles of quick clinical diagnosis, first-aid measures, decontamination techniques, and recognition of life-threatening symptoms are of primary importance. Other more theoretical aspects of toxicology may be omitted altogether or considered only briefly.

Recommendations

Clinical toxicology is still not acknowledged as a separate medical discipline in most countries. Its full acceptance as such by medical schools and the public health service is therefore desirable, and the importance of active collaboration among scientists and professionals in this area has now been internationally recognized. Every effort must be made to ensure that the relevant human resources are developed as quickly and effectively as possible. Measures to harmonize approaches to clinical toxicology throughout the world and to coordinate the work of international organizations and other international bodies in this area should be reinforced.

At the national level, the following measures should be taken to support and promote clinical toxicology:

- Clinical toxicology services should be established wherever the need for them is identified.

- The discipline of clinical toxicology should be given official recognition, as should the trained professionals who may be already working in this field.

- Academic institutions should be encouraged to develop clinical toxicology as a discipline in its own right, e.g. by establishing a department within a teaching hospital with an intensive care unit, outpatient clinic, laboratory for toxicological analysis, etc. This would be a step towards the institution of an academic career structure for clinical toxicologists.

Additional, internationally coordinated measures that would be useful in promoting clinical toxicology include the establishment of:

- mechanisms for ensuring unimpeded communication and exchange information and experience

- collaborative research projects on clinical toxicology
- international collaboration in establishing protocols for the treatment of poisoned patients and for the evaluation of antidotes
- international mechanisms for ensuring the adequate availability of antidotes and early warning of toxic hazards
- appropriate international educational programmes and exchanges.

4.
Analytical toxicology and other laboratory services

Introduction

Laboratory services are an essential component of a poison control programme. They should be capable of undertaking toxicological analyses of both biological and non-biological materials, as well as relevant biomedical analyses, on an emergency basis. In some instances this would necessitate a round-the-clock service. Each laboratory service should develop its analytical capabilities in partnership with physicians dealing with poisoning cases. Furthermore, treatment of poisoning requires cooperation between laboratory services and those who interpret the analytical data. Laboratory services also have an important role in the surveillance of populations exposed to toxic substances, e.g. rural workers exposed to pesticides.

Analytical toxicology and other laboratory services may be provided within the context of a general hospital laboratory that also conducts routine biomedical analyses but should preferably have their own specific equipment and support. A specialized analytical toxicology laboratory may also be envisaged; this would normally be associated with a multifunctional poison centre and could also provide further services to the community, such as forensic toxicology, monitoring drugs of abuse and therapeutic drugs, and biological monitoring of occupational and environmental chemical exposure.

Functions of an analytical toxicology service

The main functions of an analytical toxicology service are to provide:

- emergency qualitative and/or quantitative assays for certain common poisons, especially where knowledge of the amount of poison absorbed may influence treatment (a 24-hours-a-day service may be essential for such assays);

- more complex analyses, such as "unknown" screening for cases where the cause of illness is unknown but may involve a poison; these analyses should be available, even if not provided on an emergency basis;

- analyses to monitor the efficacy of certain treatment or elimination techniques (e.g. haemoperfusion, haemodialysis);

- analyses for the biological monitoring of populations exposed to chemicals occupationally or environmentally;

- advice on the collection, storage, and transport of specimens, and on the interpretation of results of analyses;

- research into toxicokinetics and mechanisms of toxicity, in collaboration with clinical services and poison information centres.

Depending on local circumstances, it may be cost-effective to add other functions, such as monitoring of therapeutic drugs, surveillance of drug abuse, and analysis of occupational and environmental chemicals, since these activities require similar equipment and expertise. Training is essential for staff performing toxicological analysis. A central service for analytical toxicology may provide training in the subject for other hospital laboratory staff and — for physicians who treat poisoned patients — in the interpretation of analytical data.

Location, facilities, and equipment

Location

The ideal location for an analytical toxicology laboratory is within, or close to, clinical services where poisoned patients are treated. This may facilitate the rapid transport of samples and consultation on specific cases between clinicians and analysts.

Equipment

The availability of basic equipment, including balances, centrifuges, vortex mixer, water-bath, refrigerator, freezer, and fume cupboard, is assumed. Although the analytical equipment available will inevitably depend on local requirements and circumstances, certain basic equipment for techniques such as colorimetry, spectrophotometry, and thin-layer chromatography will normally be available, even if only at the local hospital laboratory. Attention is drawn to the recent IPCS manual on simple analytical toxicological tests.[1] However, it should be emphasized that, even where the appropriate equipment is available, an experienced analytical toxicologist is still needed to provide an effective service.

The use of more sophisticated analytical techniques such as immunoassay, gas chromatography, mass spectrometry, high-performance liquid chromatography, and atomic absorption spectrophotometry requires specialized back-up facilities (servicing and consumables). A high degree of operator expertise in both the use and maintenance of such equipment is also essential. It is therefore recommended that the purchase and use of equipment for the following techniques should be undertaken only as part of a comprehensive programme for the development of analytical facilities:

simple "spot" tests
Conway apparatus
Gutzeit apparatus
direct-reading spectrophotometer
UV/visible recording spectrophotometer
thin-layer chromatography — qualitative
thin-layer chromatography — quantitative
gas chromatography — packed columns
gas chromatography — capillary columns
gas chromatography — flame ionization detection
gas chromatography — nitrogen-phosphorus detection
gas chromatography — electron-capture detection
gas chromatography — mass spectrometry
high-performance liquid chromatography — UV detection
high-performance liquid chromatography — fluorescence detection
high-performance liquid chromatography — mass spectrometry

---

[1] *Basic analytical toxicology.* Geneva, World Health Organization, 1995.

high-performance liquid chromatography — electrochemical detection
high-performance liquid chromatography — diode array UV detection
capillary electrophoresis
atomic emission spectrometry
atomic absorption spectrometry (flame)
electrothermal atomic absorption spectrometry
inductively coupled plasma source spectrometry
radioimmunoassay — counting
enzyme immunoassay (e.g. enzyme-multiplied immunoassay technique)
fluorescence immunoassay
enzyme-linked immunosorbent assay
fluorimetry
infrared spectrometry

Reference materials

The availability of pure reference compounds is essential for any analytical toxicology service. These can be purchased from some chemical suppliers or may be provided with commercial kits. In some instances, reference solutions may also be obtained from other laboratories, either locally or internationally.

Reagents and consumables

Special chemicals are required to perform many colorimetric assays and to prepare reagents for thin-layer chromatography. Particular attention should be given to ensuring a reliable supply of such chemicals. Availability of consumables for chromatographic and other techniques must be guaranteed if equipment is to be used to full advantage.

Reference works

A list of reference books on laboratory investigations is given in Section 9.

Quality assurance

The analytical data provided by laboratory services must be reliable, and this can best be ensured by employing certain basic quality assurance procedures:

- *Internal quality control.* Internal quality control involves the analysis of samples known to contain a poison of interest at the same time as clinical samples. For qualitative work, this procedure ensures the viability of the test reagents and the assay conditions. For quantitative work, specimens containing known concentrations of the poison should be analysed together with clinical samples in order to validate the procedure.

- *External quality control.* Some countries operate quality assurance programmes in which samples of known composition are regularly circulated from a central laboratory to a number of different laboratories. The receiving laboratory may be notified of the poison present and asked to determine its concentration. Alternatively, the exercise may involve the detection, identification, and subsequent measurement of unknown poison(s). Results are returned to the central coordinating laboratory and the performance of the receiving laboratory is assessed.

The training and participation of analytical toxicologists in both these aspects of quality assurance are crucial to the maintenance of good analytical performance. In addition, analysts should be made aware of, and encouraged to adopt, the principles of good laboratory practice.[1]

Safety measures

Analytical staff may be at risk both from the toxic effects of chemicals with which they work and from diseases associated with biological samples (particularly viral hepatitis B and HIV infection). Appropriate educational and safety measures are essential. Attention is drawn to a recent IUPAC/IPCS monograph dealing with the safe use and disposal of chemicals in laboratories.[2]

Staff

The staff required by a laboratory service will depend on the volume and type of toxicological and other tests to be performed, which in turn will depend on local circumstances. Every toxicological laboratory must have at least one experienced toxicological analyst and one laboratory assistant. However, a central analytical toxicology service requires a considerably larger number of staff because of the wide range of clinical and research needs it has to cover. It will also require administrative staff and possibly a documentalist.

Laboratory assistants should have been educated in one or more science subjects and have practical analytical experience such as can be gained by working in a general chemistry laboratory. The number employed will depend upon local circumstances and particular situations, such as the need to provide an emergency service. Rotation of these personnel with, for example, the staff of a local hospital laboratory could help in establishing a pool of experience. Laboratory assistants should continue in part-time education in chemistry, biochemistry, or related subjects, in addition to receiving practical in-house instruction in analytical techniques.

An analytical toxicologist should possess a university degree, or the equivalent, in chemistry, biochemistry, or a related subject such as experimental toxicology, pharmacy, or pharmacology, and have a good understanding of analytical chemistry. A further qualification, such as a doctorate, plus relevant experience that includes a high standard of practical analytical work, would be an advantage for the head of an analytical toxicology laboratory. Wider knowledge of aspects of toxicology other than analytical toxicology is also desirable. Since many basic reference works are published in English, a knowledge of that language is important. It is of paramount importance that individuals recruited for analytical toxicology posts are committed to their work; a career structure should be provided to encourage them to remain in their posts when trained and to pass their experience on to others.

The training of senior analytical toxicology staff for a central analytical toxicology service must be considered in the context of the circumstances in the country concerned. For an individual with the basic qualifications outlined in the previous paragraph, the training period would normally be a minimum of six months in total, which could be spread over several years. During this period the staff member should acquire both practical and theoretical knowledge of the following, depending on the needs of the service and the equipment and facilities available:

---

[1] *Good laboratory practice in the testing of chemicals: final report of the Group of Experts on Good Laboratory Practice.* Paris, Organisation for Economic Co-operation and Development, 1982.
[2] *Chemical safety matters.* Cambridge, Cambridge University Press, 1992.

- liquid- and solid-phase extraction techniques
- qualitative colour tests
- thin-layer chromatography
- scanning ultraviolet/visible spectrophotometry
- immunochemical assays (radioimmunoassay, enzyme-multiplied immunoassay, fluorescence polarization immunoassay)
- gas chromatography (flame ionization, electron capture, and nitrogen/phosphorus detection)
- high-performance liquid chromatography
- mass spectrometry
- flame and electrothermal atomic absorption spectrophotometry
- toxicokinetics, metabolism, and human toxicology of the substances analysed, with emphasis on the interpretation of results
- basic pathology as far as this relates to clinical toxicology
- laboratory management (choice, handling, and storage of specimens, reporting and recording of results)
- good laboratory practice and quality assurance procedures
- teaching and oral presentation of cases and reviews of the literature and the results of research projects.

Wherever possible, the training should lead to a recognized diploma. The analyst will continue to gain practical on-the-job experience, particularly as the work of the analytical toxicology service expands. Continuing education, such as participation in research and development projects, case presentations, and attendance at international meetings, should be encouraged. Membership of national and international toxicological and pharmacological societies should also be encouraged.

Table 3
Criteria for laboratories providing training in clinical analytical toxicology

Staff
- The laboratory should be headed by a toxicologist with at least 5 years' experience in clinical analytical toxicology. In addition, he or she should have suitable academic qualifications (e.g. a doctorate), have published original research, and have teaching experience.

- At least two experienced analytical toxicologists should also work in the laboratory to ensure comprehensive coverage.

Organization
- The laboratory should offer a 24-hour emergency service and should be associated with a multifunctional poison centre providing an information service and patient care, so as to facilitate contact between the clinical and analytical services.

- A wide range of analyses should be available on a regular basis and it should be possible to undertake special investigations according to needs (e.g. occupational exposure to toxic metals and certain pesticides; monitoring of drug use).

Techniques
- Instruction in the following techniques should be readily available:

    — qualitative colour tests
    — thin-layer chromatography
    — scanning ultraviolet/visible spectrophotometry
    — immunochemical assays (radioimmunoassay, enzyme-multiplied immunoassay, fluorescence polarization immunoassay)
    — gas-liquid chromatography (flame ionization, electron capture, nitrogen/phosphorus detection)
    — high-performance liquid chromatography (ultraviolet, fluorescence, electrochemical detection)
    — flame and electrothermal atomic absorption spectrophotometry
    — liquid- and solid-phase extraction techniques.

The training required by the head of a laboratory will also depend on local circumstances. If a country does not yet have a suitable training programme, help should be sought from countries with well established analytical toxicology services, which should be encouraged to provide training fellowships. In a country that already has an analytical toxicology service, but needs additional expertise in particular fields, visiting experts from other countries may be invited to provide the necessary training. Sample criteria for laboratories providing training in analytical toxicology are given in Table 3.

Laboratory staff should be encouraged to participate in regular meetings within a multifunctional poison control centre in order to:

- review case reports and, in particular, discuss the medical interpretation of analytical results with the clinical personnel

- review developments in analytical toxicology published in the literature

- examine results of research carried out in the laboratory and identify areas for cooperative investigation or further research

- discuss laboratory management in relation to the overall work on poison control.

Laboratory staff should also be encouraged to present papers at, and participate in, scientific meetings of relevance to their work.

5.

Toxicovigilance and prevention of poisoning

Introduction

Poison information centres have a fundamental role, in partnership with others, in toxicovigilance and prevention. Toxicovigilance consists of the active observation and evaluation of toxic risks and phenomena in the community — an activity that should result in measures aimed to reduce or remove risks. Thus its main goal is prevention.

The role of poison information centres in toxicovigilance includes:

- identifying serious poisoning risks in the local community, and the substances, circumstances, and population groups involved;

- identifying changes in the incidence of poisoning, e.g. different substances of abuse, application of new pesticides, and seasonal variations in the incidence of poisoning, such as carbon monoxide poisoning from heating appliances;

- monitoring the toxicity of commercial products, such as household, industrial, and agricultural chemicals, as well as pharmaceuticals (by any route of administration), for acute, medium-term, and chronic effects, with particular regard to new products and formulations (e.g. overuse of analgesics, occupational exposure to solvents);

- monitoring the toxic effects of drug overdosage;

- identifying substances that cause significant morbidity and mortality, and specific effects on target organs (e.g. high incidence of renal insufficiency, fetal malformations);

- reporting to health authorities and other relevant bodies situations that demand preventive or corrective action, and, where appropriate, calling an alert;

- monitoring the effectiveness of preventive measures.

Where new or altered patterns of poisoning are identified by centres, the data should be strictly verified and evaluated before they are reported to those in charge of community health and regulatory actions and/or to the manufacturers or users of the chemicals involved. Sometimes, this information should also be disseminated at the international level, notably to other poison information centres, professional bodies concerned with toxicology, and organizations such as WHO.

Preventive measures for both individual and multiple cases of poisoning should be established on the basis of the available data on high-risk factors, particularly the circumstances, the substances involved, and the potential victims.

A centre could initiate its preventive activities by reporting information on toxic hazards, identified by toxicovigilance, to those with the authority to take appropriate action, and by giving information and advice to those involved in health education. Further preventive activities could include educational campaigns, producing educational material, and planning, in partnership with others, the implementation and evaluation of preventive measures.

The principal types of preventive action that should be initiated by poison information centres are:

- education, which is a most important part of any action and should be aimed at particular groups at risk, as well as the general public and professional health care workers;

- reports to, and collaboration with, various organizations and institutions on such matters as the development of safer products, safety measures relating to the packaging, design, labelling, transport, and handling of hazardous products, and withdrawing or limiting the availability of selected toxic substances.

Collaboration among all partners in a poison control programme should be strengthened in order to enhance the efficacy of toxicovigilance and preventive actions. The essential partners are:

- poison information centres, facilities for toxicological analysis, and clinical toxicology services, which have a key role in identifying and studying toxicological risks and problems;

- medical and paramedical professionals, such as hospital physicians, general practitioners, occupational physicians, coroners and medico-legal experts, psychiatrists, and pharmacists, all of whom are in a position to collect data that supplement and complement those generated by poison information centres;

- government and local authorities, which have the power to ban or control the use of high-risk chemicals;

- industries, including manufacturers, transporters, and users of chemicals, who should provide the necessary data on the chemicals they handle and cooperate in the implementation of preventive measures;

- universities and research institutions, particularly those concerned with experimental clinical toxicology, which may provide valuable data on chemicals and contribute to their identification and control;

- specialists in mass communications and sociologists, who, in the event of a toxicological emergency, should advise on the appropriate message to the public and its dissemination in a manner that will avoid misunderstandings and alarmism.

Toxicovigilance and prevention programmes

Depending on the facilities that exist in a particular country, minimum programmes for toxicovigilance and prevention should be established initially, with the aim of expanding them later. Such programmes require good basic information about the local situation, including details of acute and chronic poisoning cases, problems of environmental contamination, drug abuse, and circumstances in which there is a high risk of exposure.

Priority should be given to collecting this minimum basic data, which can be done cheaply and reasonably quickly by using:

- data from enquiries received by the poison information centre, which may provide valuable qualitative and quantitative information on cases of poisoning and be used for the evaluation of preventive activities;

- case data from accident and emergency wards, forensic departments, and local hospitals or occupational health clinics;

- technical information on toxic products and their effects, which can be obtained from the literature and other direct sources such as manufacturers and importers of chemicals.

The data collected should permit the identification of local populations at risk and of harmful substances and dangerous circumstances that are likely to play a part in local poisoning cases. This should be helpful for planning appropriate preventive measures.

Documentary resources and other facilities

The minimum documentary resources and physical facilities required are the following:

- textbooks, reviews, manuals, periodicals, and other scientific publications, which would normally be available in poison information centres and which are mostly supplied by medical libraries, manufacturers, importers, and health authorities;

- selected references and periodicals concerning the local situation and needs;

- analysed data on enquiries received by the poison information centre;

- reports of surveys and monitoring carried out by other poison information centres;

- educational material produced by other poison information centres;

- suitable space for conferences and educational events;

- office supplies and equipment;

- simple means for reproducing leaflets and hand-outs.

For maximum effectiveness, however, a programme for toxicovigilance and prevention of poisoning must have comprehensive data on all chemical substances and natural toxins found in the country concerned and appropriate evaluated case data on poisoning (with specific and detailed treatment procedures). Among the additional facilities required are the following:

- statistical and epidemiological data
- a specialized library
- communication facilities, with equipment for monitoring and recording calls
- access to computerized databases
- computers for storage and retrieval of data
- facilities for microfilming
- educational and instructional materials (brochures, posters, slides, videotapes) and facilities for producing them
- space for information resources, data storage, staff administration, and public and professional education.

Staff

A minimum programme for toxicovigilance and the prevention of poisoning requires staff with toxicological training and experience. For a full-scale programme, the poison information centre would need, in addition to those running the telephone enquiry service and dealing with patients, a sufficient number of people to follow up enquiries, write reports, and design and implement preventive activities. Training in epidemiology and the use of statistics is highly valuable in view of the type of studies required for toxicovigilance. Staff involved should be familiar with the legislation and regulations concerning the safety of chemical products and be aware of local toxicological problems related to the environment and to veterinary medicine. They should also be taught how to deal with the public, the mass media, and professionals from other fields in order to communicate the message of prevention.

The director of the centre should also:

- have some knowledge of other disciplines relevant to toxicovigilance and the prevention of poisoning;

- be able to supervise the analysis of data and promote epidemiological research;

- ensure that a periodic (at least annual) assessment is made of the evolution of poisoning problems in the country or region concerned and that the relevant authorities are kept informed about preventive measures;

- utilize available data to call an alert on toxicological problems when necessary, enlist the cooperation of relevant partners, and plan effective action;

- ensure that adequate educational material on the prevention of poisoning is prepared for both health care professionals and the public, including material for use in paediatric outpatient clinics, by teachers and children at school, and by doctors in rural hospitals;

- identify sources of funding for preventive activities (e.g. for the publication of colourful, easily understood brochures or posters, and for financing campaigns and educational courses).

Besides the staff of poison information centres, other specialists who should be involved in toxicovigilance and prevention include:

- *health educators* to design programmes, contact the mass media, and supervise effective continuous distribution of educational material;

- *primary health workers* to promote prevention at community level;

- *psychiatrists* to evaluate the incidence and severity of certain types of poisoning (e.g. in suicide attempts) in order to study the possibilities of preventing or minimizing them;

- *social workers* to evaluate the social conditions that may be determinants in some types of poisoning case, and to advise on ways of getting clear messages to target populations;

- *experimental toxicologists* to provide experimental data on chemicals and their properties.

Toxicovigilance and poisoning prevention programmes also need the support of adequate administrative and secretarial personnel.

Recommendations

The efficacy of toxicovigilance and of measures for the prevention of poisoning could be considerably enhanced by the implementation of a number of measures at both national and international level.

Recommended action at national level

Efficient communication and coordination between all partners in a poison control programme are primary ingredients for the development of effective national plans for toxicovigilance and prevention. As part of a long-term strategy, adequate knowledge of local poisoning cases should be assembled through data collection and epidemiological investigations. Computerization should facilitate the storage, handling, and rapid analysis of the data. It is therefore essential to promote:

- a system for the centralized registration of poisoned patients treated in hospitals (with diagnostic codes), together with mechanisms for the follow-up of patients in order to identify and evaluate possible medium- and long-term sequelae;

- regulations for the notification of poisoning incidents (e.g. obligatory anonymous reporting of all cases);

- the collection of sound morbidity and mortality statistics with precise certification of death by cause (e.g. from public health systems and forensic departments);

- the pooling of information collected from related areas of mutual interest, e.g. experimental toxicology, analytical toxicology, occupational medicine;

- contacts with industry for the exchange of information on chemical products manufactured and used, and the circumstances and effects of poisoning by these chemicals.

Official support for, and recognition of, the role of poison information centres in toxicovigilance and prevention of poisoning would add weight to the preventive actions instituted by a centre and make it easier for a centre to obtain complete data on the composition of toxic and potentially toxic products. In some cases, legislation providing for the confidential disclosure of the chemical composition of products to poison information centres would be of great value. Legislative authorities should seek the recommendations and advice of poison information centres concerning control measures and legislation to prevent poisoning.

Preventive and educational action may be aimed at the whole community (for example, campaigns for the prevention of poisoning, posters demonstrating the dangers of poisoning by household products and how to avoid them, booklets showing how to recognize poisonous fungi and plants) or specific groups at risk (e.g. on such subjects as pharmaceuticals and pregnancy, the safe use of pesticides by rural workers, and the risks of self-medication in the elderly). Media and communications experts have a vital role in preventive action, since the messages employed should be concise, clearly understandable, and attractive.

The methods employed for preventing, and generating awareness about, poisoning should be adapted to suit national situations and circumstances.

Recommended action at international level

In any country, the problems arising from chemical poisoning are closely linked to geographical, climatic, demographic, economic, and sociocultural conditions. However, tens of thousands of chemicals are in commercial use, and the same chemicals, drugs, or natural toxins may be found in quite different domestic or working environments in different countries, and as contaminants of air, soil, and water. Products containing these chemicals are widely traded throughout the world, and the movement of environmental contaminants does not respect national frontiers.

Many chemicals "travel" when carried by people (e.g. as medicines obtained on holidays, drugs of abuse, insect repellents), and, if unavailable or not in commercial use in a particular country, may be unknown to the local poison information centre. Co-operation between poison information centres in different countries, and with international organizations, may be of value to both national and international programmes for toxicovigilance and the prevention of poisoning.

Poison information centres may arrange to share data on toxic risks, which would permit early warning of potential problems. Pooling of information and expertise in respect of case data on rare, limited, or new phenomena, and of substance data on new hazardous products may enable preventive measures to be taken at an early stage. For the useful exchange of information, it is also essential for collaborators to standardize terminology, agreeing on matters of format and content as well as on the procedures involved in the exchange.

The following are recognized as areas in which international collaboration, through organizations such as IPCS and the World Federation, is needed:

- the exchange between poison information centres and the relevant authorities of bibliographies and documentation on internationally traded formulated products, or on products found outside their country of origin;

- the establishment of centralized or regional systems for the collection and exchange of data on poisoning cases, including their follow-up, and for the assessment, validation, analysis, and storage of these data;

- the establishment of a mechanism for the rapid notification of toxic alerts called in any country and the exchange of experience in dealing with such alerts;

- the exchange of experience of education and training programmes in the field of toxicovigilance and prevention of poisoning;

- the production and dissemination of educational materials on the prevention of poisoning, including material targeted at specific high-risk groups, to be adapted by each centre for local use.

6.

Response to major emergencies involving chemicals[1]

Introduction

The accidental discharge of chemicals during industrial operations, as well as during transport by land, sea, and inland waterways, is a growing problem throughout the world. Chemical accidents do not always involve cases of poisoning. However, people exposed to a major release of chemicals may, in some instances, be seriously contaminated and require emergency treatment. Chemical discharge may pollute the environment and give rise to poisoning in populations some distance from the accident itself. Major incidents involving many cases of poisoning may also be caused by the accidental or deliberate contamination of food, water, medicines, or consumer goods by synthetic chemicals or natural toxins. In some cases, these incidents may not be immediately associated with chemical contamination but are identified through the toxicovigilance activities of poison information centres.

Many countries have emergency plans covering the fullest possible range of natural and technological disasters. The fire and rescue services, together with the police, are usually the first to be involved in the response to a major chemical accident. By providing appropriate information, poison information centres have an important contribution to make to the handling of major incidents involving chemicals, and clinical toxicology services may also be involved in the treatment of victims. Centres should take an active part in contingency planning, education, and training for chemical accidents. They should also initiate research and follow-up studies when appropriate. A poison information centre often has the advantage of being the only centre of its kind in a country or a region providing a 24-hours-a-day service and may therefore play a central role in chemical emergencies.

The staff of the poison information centre should receive specific instructions on how to act in the case of a chemical disaster. They should be prepared to provide relevant information on the chemicals involved to those responsible for handling the emergency or alert procedures, as well as to decision-makers and the mass media. They should know how to recognize the magnitude or level of the accident (whether it is operational, local, regional, or international) and should alert the centre's director, other staff, and health and other authorities, according to established procedures.

Staff must also be trained to deal with the general public, either directly or, preferably, through the mass media. They should be instructed on how to avoid creating panic and how to communicate calmly with others involved in responding to the disaster and also with the community, providing reassurance and a clear message. Retrospective studies of chemical incidents that have occurred in the area or examination of hypothetical disaster situations may form a good basis for the training of staff and for contingency planning with other concerned bodies.

---

[1] See also: *Health aspects of chemical accidents. Guidance on chemical accident awareness, preparedness and response for health professionals and emergency responders*. Paris, Organisation for Economic Co-operation and Development, 1994 (OCDE/GD (94)1).

Information

The poison information centre may act as the focal point for action in case of chemical accidents and should be prepared to provide adequate information rapidly in the acute phases. When building up toxicological data banks, centres should therefore include information on all chemicals likely to be involved in accidents in the region, not forgetting the less frequently used industrial chemicals and reactive intermediates. It is important to have information on:

- toxic chemicals and their effects
- high-risk areas and processes and/or activities involving risk
- which chemical(s) might be released, in what forms and quantities
- possible protective and remedial measures.

The exact location, capabilities, and capacities of treatment and toxicological analytical services and of facilities for emergency transport must be known. Centres must also be aware of the responsibilities and roles of all bodies involved in contingency planning, and establish close communication links with rescue services and the police. The information may have to be gathered by the poison information centre itself if emergency contingency planning has not yet been organized in the country or may be requested from the authorities when such plans exist and are operative. There is often a legal requirement for authorities to be notified of highly hazardous activities involving the use of chemicals and of the location of stored chemicals; such information could valuably be made available to poison information centres as well. In some countries, poison information centres, identified as focal points for chemical disasters, are informed when dangerous cargoes are being transported or high-risk manoeuvres involving toxic chemicals are to be undertaken in the areas they serve.

Experience with industrial accidents involving chemicals is often available at the plants concerned but not always elsewhere. It is of vital importance for poison information centres to have access to this experience, and for activities that encourage exchanges of information and experience between different occupational health services and poison information centres to be established.

In the event of a major chemical accident, poison information centres may expect a flood of telephone calls. They should be prepared to deal with this type of situation, avoiding panic and providing advice rapidly to all concerned parties.

Treatment

Staff at clinical toxicology services may be involved in the treatment of victims of chemical incidents or disasters. They need to provide guidance to the medical rescue teams on the triage of poisoned patients, on their initial treatment procedures before they reach hospital, and on decontamination at the site of the incident. Any hospital that treats patients may need to provide decontamination facilities outside its emergency admission area in order to prevent contamination of the hospital by toxic chemicals.

Contingency planning

Poison information centres should cooperate with other agencies in contingency planning for chemical accidents. Some countries, especially the more highly industrialized, have coordinated contingency plans in which a number of specific activities are demanded of poison information centres. In the many countries that lack an established emergency response system the responsibility of poison information centres may be even greater: they may suddenly be obliged to assume responsibility for the handling of an emergency. If contingency plans have already been established, a poison information centre may become an emergency control centre in the event of a chemical disaster. New centres should therefore have the foresight to consider what chemical disasters could occur within their region and be prepared to provide fast, accurate advice and orientation.

Emergency medical plans must be extended to cover chemical accidents, and close collaboration should be established between the planners and the poison information centre. The centre should provide the planners with guidelines on: measures for risk assessment; decontamination *in situ* and within hospitals; first-aid measures; general and specific therapy; and measures to ensure the availability of antidotes. At the medical level, poison information centres should also be aware of the facilities available for dealing with large numbers of victims in terms of number of beds, pharmaceutical supplies, and availability of specific antidotes.

Education and training

Poison information centres should play an active role in the education and training of all members of rescue teams for their role in the event of chemical accidents. This education and training should be geared to the educational level of each group being trained (e.g. firemen, field commanders, supervisors, telephone and radio operators, doctors). Training should cover decontamination techniques and protective measures for medical staff treating contaminated patients, as well as triage techniques.

Follow-up studies

Close follow-up studies of both major and minor chemical accidents may yield much valuable information on their handling. In the event of a major incident involving chemicals, poison information centres should be ready to mobilize competent personnel. Appropriate data on the accident should be collected to enable exposure to be related to clinical features of poisoning. This requires preparation in advance. A staff member from the centre may need to go to the scene of the incident, or to the place where the patients are being treated, in order to take an active part in evaluation and risk assessment, coordinate advice to health care personnel on site, and organize analytical tests. This would also provide an opportunity to collect human toxicological data, valuable for advice on future occasions and for further planning in respect of chemical accidents.

Financial support

If poison information centres are to respond adequately to major incidents involving chemicals, financial support may be required from the government. Personnel from the centres should have the opportunity to participate in educational activities and visit the sites of accidents outside their own areas in order to gather relevant information and experience. This is important not only during the acute phase of an incident but also at later stages when conclusions can be drawn from the incident and recommendations made.

Collaboration between centres

The need for close national and international collaboration between poison information centres is recognized. The hazards arising from the manufacture, storage, and transport of chemicals are sometimes shared by neighbouring countries, in which case concerted action should be taken to prevent or reduce the likelihood and impact of chemical accidents. Poison information centres should therefore undertake periodic exchanges of information on high-risk circumstances for chemical accidents, and be consulted concerning relevant international or intergovernmental agreements.

To assist in the identification of chemicals to which an individual may have been exposed, it is essential for a poison information centre to build up a database of relevant information on commercial and other local products found in the area it serves. A simple card file can be used for this purpose. Alternatively, if a centre is contemplating computerization of its database, the IPCS INTOX format for standardizing product information (see Annex 4) is recommended.

7.

Antidotes and their availability

Introduction

Antidotes may play an important role in the treatment of poisoning. While good supportive care and elimination techniques may, in many cases, restore a poisoned patient to good health and stabilize his or her body functions, the appropriate use of antidotes and other agents may greatly enhance elimination and counteract the toxic actions of the poison. In certain circumstances they may significantly reduce the medical resources otherwise needed to treat a patient, shorten the period of therapy, and, in some cases, save a patient from death. Thus, antidotes may sometimes reduce the overall burden on the health service of managing cases of poisoning. In areas remote from good hospital services, and particularly in developing countries that lack adequate facilities for supportive care, antidotes may be even more essential in the treatment of poisoning.

Physicians frequently express concern about the difficulty of obtaining certain antidotes in an emergency. The IPCS and the EC, in consultation with the World Federation, are undertaking a project designed to evaluate the efficacy of antidotes and to encourage their availability. In a preparatory phase of this project an antidote was defined as a therapeutic substance used to counteract the toxic action(s) of a specified xenobiotic. A preliminary list of antidotes, and of other agents used to prevent the absorption of poisons, to enhance their elimination, and to counteract their effects on body functions, was established; preliminary classification of these agents was based on urgency of treatment and efficacy in practice. Agents that correspond to the WHO concept of an essential drug were designated as such, and some have already been incorporated into the WHO List of Essential Drugs.[1] Antidotes and substances for veterinary use were also listed. Methods and principles for the evaluation of antidotes and other agents used in the treatment of poisoning were drafted and are being used as a framework for preparing monographs on specific antidotes, which are being published in a special series.[2]

Early in the course of this preparatory work, it became apparent that the availability of antidotes differed from one country to another. A survey of selected poison information centres was undertaken in order to identify the specific difficulties experienced in obtaining antidotes. Results showed that poison centres in industrialized countries generally have few problems in obtaining most antidotes, although administrative difficulties and the lack of suitable preparations and of importers and manufacturers hinder access to certain antidotes. Centres in developing countries, however, reported many problems in obtaining even the common antidotes that are readily available elsewhere. Problems generally arose in the following three interrelated areas:

---

[1] *The use of essential drugs. Model List of Essential Drugs (ninth list). Seventh report of the WHO Expert Committee.* Geneva, World Health Organization, 1997 (WHO Technical Report Series, No. 867).

[2] *IPCS/EC Evaluation of antidotes.* Cambridge, Cambridge University Press.

- scientific, technical, and economic considerations
- regulatory and administrative requirements
- considerations of time and geography

Scientific aspects

The efficacy of a substance used as an antidote must be scientifically validated, initially through animal experiments, preferably using species that exhibit a pattern of toxicity similar to that in humans. The clinical efficacy of an antidote in humans may be more difficult to ascertain and document than that of other pharmaceutical agents, since there is little opportunity for clinical trials. The potential toxicity of an antidote is important in deciding its use, and the possibility of adverse reactions should always be considered. An antidote known to be non-toxic may be used in cases of poisoning even if its efficacy is uncertain; a toxic antidote, however, should be used only if its therapeutic effect is known and the diagnosis certain. Adverse effects and chronic toxicity may be less important than in the case of an ordinary pharmaceutical agent, since an antidote is likely to be used only once. It is important that increased toxicity does not result from mobilization of the toxic substance from tissue stores or from changes in tissue distribution, as in the case of the transient rise in blood levels of lead, and precipitation of acute encephalopathy, after inappropriate use of antidotes in children.

The importance of full validation of the efficacy of substances to be used as antidotes must be emphasized.

Improved knowledge of the mechanisms of toxicity of different poisons and of the kinetics of toxic substances may also facilitate the development and use of specific antidotes. Once an effective antidote has been identified, there remains the problem of its manufacture as a pharmaceutical substance suitable for use in humans. The formulation of a preparation for oral use will, in many cases, make it easier to administer the antidote, for example in ambulatory patients.

The scientific study of antidotes thus has implications for drug regulation authorities and governments, for the commercial sector, and for poison information centres.

- *Drug regulation authorities and governments.* Comprehensive scientific studies will enable regulatory authorities to facilitate the registration of useful, effective antidotes. Governments are responsible for ensuring the availability of antidotes and should recognize the importance of this group of therapeutic agents and the need to support their scientific study.

- *The commercial sector.* The manufacture and supply of antidotes are usually the responsibility of the commercial sector, which may also need to support appropriate studies. Industries involved in the manufacture and supply of potentially toxic agents must consider their possible effects on users and on others who may be exposed; they should ensure that appropriate antidotes are available on the local market.

- *Poison information centres.* Poison information centres, and especially the treatment units, have an essential role in monitoring the use of antidotes. Ideally, data on antidote use should be collected in an internationally standardized manner to allow results to be compared and recommendations made. International exchange of information should be encouraged to allow critical assessment of the efficacy and side-effects of antidotal agents. Health care professionals should be aware that the data required at the time certain antidotes were registered may have been quite limited and may therefore need updating in the light of more recent findings.

Even an effective and readily available antidote will be useless if the attending physician is unable to establish a correct diagnosis or is uninformed about the availability or indications for use of the antidote. Information programmes should be arranged by toxicological and poison information centres in order to familiarize clinical personnel with the proper use of antidotes, particularly for individuals in high-risk groups, such as those exposed to hazardous chemicals in the course of their work.

Technical aspects

Registration

Registration of a pharmaceutical for use as an antidote would seem a satisfactory means of dealing with problems of distribution and availability. However, some pharmaceutical manufacturers are disinclined to register antidotes because of the small volume of production required to meet market demand. It is therefore suggested that a means should be found of encouraging industries that market potentially toxic drugs or chemicals to provide information on antidotal treatment, and to facilitate the provision and registration of appropriate antidotes. Pharmaceutical companies that produce antidotes should be encouraged to register them in their countries of use. It would also be helpful to ease the administrative procedures required to permit the use of an antidote — for example by making it an "orphan drug"[1] or a "common drug" for which the registration procedure is less complicated (see page 57).

Chemicals as antidotes

Some chemical substances with antidotal properties, for example calcium chloride, sodium nitrite, and methylene blue, are marketed as chemicals but are not available in appropriate formulations for use as drugs. It is therefore important to ensure that the quality and purity of these chemicals will permit their administration as antidotes. Pharmacopoeia commissions should consider issuing monographs on such chemicals.

Formulation of antidotes

Certain pharmaceutical agents may be registered for uses other than as antidotes and are thus not available in appropriate formulations, or in adequate quantities, to meet the needs of poisoned patients. Additional authorization for use of these agents as specific antidotes should not present a major problem, but the necessary procedures need to be facilitated.

National distribution of antidotes

Demographic, geographical, and economic factors sometimes hinder the availability of antidotes. In addition, the high cost that results from infrequent demand and short shelf-life may prevent their widespread distribution. A central "bank" of antidotes could be an economic and effective means of ensuring distribution, and this should be

---

[1] Orphan drugs: drugs for diseases or conditions that occur so infrequently that there is no reasonable expectation of the costs of developing and marketing being recovered through revenues from sales. The United States Government provides incentives for the production of such drugs, including tax credits, seven-year exclusive rights, facility in the Food and Drug Administration registration process, and a financial grant to cover part of the clinical research.

organized by health authorities in such a way that any poison victim may be assured of receiving an antidote within the appropriate period of time.

Economic aspects

When considering the cost of antidotes, governments should take into account the social and medical consequences of failure to treat poisoned patients in an appropriate manner and the continued economic burden on local or national resources that may ensue.

In general, pharmaceutical companies will manufacture and supply antidotes only if they are encouraged by adequate economic returns for their investment and by simple registration procedures. To this end, governments should consider recent WHO recommendations[1] concerning products for export and facilitate the registration of antidotes already evaluated and registered elsewhere.

If antidotes cannot be supplied by the pharmaceutical industry, other means of ensuring their availability should be considered. These could include the establishment of government manufacturing facilities, a manufacturing pharmacy laboratory, or a system that allows the importation of antidotes registered elsewhere.

Other ways of using resources efficiently, such as rationalizing the purchase and distribution of antidotes, should also be considered by health authorities and should take into account the time within which antidotes need to be available for use in treatment. Local transport conditions should also be considered (see page 58).

Registration and administrative requirements

Antidotes are pharmaceutical products, and almost all countries have an official body concerned with the registration and approval of pharmaceutical substances. Many antidotes are drugs that have undergone a full range of tests before registration and are authorized for distribution and use in many countries. Such tests usually cover the physicochemical properties, stability of the formulation, and toxicity as determined by animal experiments, pharmacological studies, and clinical trials. However, certain pharmaceutical agents that have been evaluated for other uses may require additional authorization for antidotal use. This type of registration should present no major problem and could follow the procedure for a new antidote referred to in the next paragraph. There may, however, be a need to develop special formulations to allow sufficient quantities to be available for administration as an antidote.

For a new pharmaceutical substance to be used *only* as an antidote, the registration procedure could be modified so that it is less comprehensive than that for a normal drug. Authorities often accept different criteria for the registration of certain pharmaceutical substances, for example anticancer drugs, because of the special conditions that apply to their use. A new antidote could be considered in a similar light, thereby facilitating its registration and encouraging manufacturers to make it more widely available.

As already mentioned, a number of chemical substances that are not strictly pharmaceutical products, such as calcium chloride, sodium nitrite, and methylene blue, may

---

[1] *WHO Expert Committee on Specifications for Pharmaceutical Preparations. Thirty-fourth report.* Geneva, World Health Organization, 1996 (WHO Technical Report Series, No. 863): Section 6.2, The WHO Certification Scheme on the Quality of Pharmaceutical Products Moving in International Commerce.

be used as antidotes. If they are to be made available for administration to poisoned patients, their quality and purity become important considerations.

Some antidotes that have been registered and approved in individual countries, after extensive testing, are faced with trade or administrative barriers when their importation into other countries is considered; examples include activated charcoal, syrup of ipecacuanha, and oximes. Countries should select from the list of essential antidotes (see Annex 2) those agents that are most appropriate to their needs; in some cases, these drugs are already listed in the WHO List of Essential Drugs.[1]

In some countries, existing regulations may inhibit the use of certain substances — for example, antidotes still undergoing clinical trial and not yet registered — in the treatment of poisoning, even when these substances would be of value in clinically oriented poison control centres. Special legal provision should be made for practising physicians in clinical toxicology and poison control centres to use these agents — particularly in "life-saving" circumstances — on the basis of their own judgement. In addition, it should be possible to stock these substances under controlled conditions at poison control centres and to exchange them between such centres. These measures would encourage the interchange of experience and improve the database for subsequent registration. It is important, though, that a mechanism be established to ensure the purity and sterility of unregistered antidotal agents.

Considerations of time and geography

The availability of an antidote is highly dependent on its distribution within a country as well as its source, particularly if it has to be imported from another country. The best way of ensuring the importation of antidotes into a country might be to entrust it entirely to a central organization or institution. The establishment of a central agency responsible for the importation and distribution of antidotes is therefore recommended; alternatively, the task could be entrusted to clinically oriented poison control centres.

Many countries already have such centralized systems for the importation of pharmaceutical agents. It is essential for the institutions concerned to consult and cooperate with national poison control and clinical toxicology centres, or associations of such centres, so that the importation of antidotes reflects local needs. Where certain antidotes are not available, either from local manufacturers or as imports, the central institution may cooperate with poison centres in recommending their local manufacture by hospital pharmacies or through pharmaceutical associations. Furthermore, in the event of an emergency or chemical disaster, an exchange arrangement between poison centres in different countries might make it possible to obtain a supply of some antidotes that are commercially available elsewhere.

Since many antidotes are expensive, infrequently used, and have a limited shelf-life, central stocking of antidotes makes sound economic sense; it makes inspection easier and ensures a supply of products that have not lost their effectiveness. However, any such centralized system must be able to guarantee that a poisoned patient will receive an antidote within the time required for treatment. Certain agents used in the treatment of poisoning, for example, syrup of ipecacuanha and activated charcoal, are used frequently; others are required for use immediately, e.g. those used in the treatment of cyanide poisoning. Antidotes have been classified as those needed:

---

[1] *The use of essential drugs. Model List of Essential Drugs (ninth list). Seventh report of the WHO Expert Committee.* Geneva; World Health Organization, 1997 (WHO Technical Report Series, No. 867).

- immediately (within 30 minutes)
- within 2 hours
- within 6 hours.

Antidotes needed immediately must be stocked at all hospitals, as well as in health centres or doctors' surgeries if the nearest hospital is some distance away. It may also be necessary to have certain antidotes available at places of work for use under medical supervision (e.g. in factories using cyanide). Antidotes needed within 2 hours can be stocked at certain main hospitals; patients can be taken to these hospitals for treatment or the antidotes can be transported — within the time limit — to the health facilities at which treatment is provided. Antidotes needed within 6 hours may be stocked at central regional depots, provided that there are adequate facilities for transporting them within the time limit. For all categories of antidotes, there is the further option of keeping a small amount, sufficient to start treatment, in stock locally, further supplies being obtained from a central source as required.

Where certain types of poisoning are frequent, or in areas where certain chemicals are heavily used, the appropriate antidotes may be kept in ambulances, operated by physicians, that are sent out to treat cases of poisoning. Poisoning by natural toxins may be seasonal and may be specific to certain regions (e.g. snake-bites in rural areas during planting and harvesting seasons). Antivenoms may be sent to rural areas during these seasons to be readily available in case of need. The rapid transport of antidotes may be needed in certain cirumstances, and appropriate advance arrangements should be made, e.g. for the use of official cars, aircraft, or trains. In certain situations, arrangements for the rapid transport of patients to hospitals with appropriate facilities and antidotes may be necessary. Comprehensive instructions on interim treatment measures should be given to first-aid workers or other medical or paramedical professionals.

In deciding where antidotes should be stocked, a number of factors should be taken into consideration, notably the following:

- the size of the country and the area to be covered by a depot
- the density of the population
- the incidence of poisonings that require special therapeutic measures and/or antidotes
- the social and economic activities of the region that may be associated with a high risk of poisoning
- the distances of hospitals and health centres from the depot
- communications (road, air services, etc.) between the depot and the hospitals or health centres
- the cost of antidotes and of the wastage caused by expiry of effectiveness compared with the cost of transport in case of emergency.

The most logical location for a regional central depot is a poison information centre or central hospital pharmacy. The economic management of the supply of antidotes could be improved by a central, preferably computerized, record system, regularly updated. The need to hold contingency stocks of antidotes for response to chemical disasters should be considered, especially in areas where large amounts of potentially hazardous chemicals are being manufactured, used, transported or stored. There, regional cooperation between centres, permitting the exchange of information on the availability of antidotes, is highly desirable.

The conditions under which antidotes are stored are important determinants of their maximum shelf-life and an essential consideration when storage depots are chosen.

Greater efforts should be made to find antidotes with longer shelf-lives and improved stability under harsh conditions, particularly of temperature and humidity, for use in areas where proper storage cannot be achieved.

Special problems of developing countries

In addition to the general problems of availability discussed above, it is recognized that developing countries may have special problems as regards antidotes. Many of these countries do not have poison information centres and lack the facilities available in developed countries for supportive treatment of poisoning. Consequently, they may have a greater need for certain antidotes, for example naloxone. It is important that these countries should establish centres to provide the relevant information, to recommend, whenever appropriate, the use of antidotes, and to coordinate the distribution of antidotes.

Health authorities are sometimes unable or reluctant to facilitate the import of antidotes, since the procedures involved may be cumbersome and lengthy. Economic problems, including a shortage of convertible currency, are liable to worsen the situation. The pattern of poisoning in any given country should indicate the extent of the need to facilitate registration procedures and to acquire particular antidotes.

Good first-aid procedures and the appropriate use of antidotes may be not only life-saving but also economically sound. Although antidotes are sometimes expensive, their use may prevent death, prolonged hospitalization, or permanent sequelae. The benefits of their use thus outweigh the costs. International agencies may be helpful in enabling some countries to acquire the antidotes they need.

Lack of adequate communication systems and transport infrastructure in certain countries may make it impossible to transport antidotes sufficiently quickly in an emergency. Measures to ensure the rapid transport of antidotes to affected areas, or, alternatively, the transport of poisoned patients to appropriate treatment facilities, are therefore of the greatest importance. It may be difficult to find adequate facilities for emergency storage depots; furthermore, local conditions and climate may make routine storage of antidotes difficult in certain areas of the country. Nevertheless, it is essential to ensure correct storage, and due account should be taken of expiry dates and the necessary conditions of temperature, light, and humidity. Proper storage conditions are also essential during the transportation of antidotes from the point of importation to local depots, and in transitional storage areas.

Antidotes for veterinary use

Poisoning in animals is a serious problem in many parts of the world, and poison information centres often receive enquiries regarding the treatment of poisoned animals. The use of antidotes in veterinary medicine poses a number of special problems as regards choice, dosage, route of administration, and availability. It is therefore recommended that each country should make separate arrangements for the examination of various aspects of veterinary use of antidotes by a working group with the necessary expertise, which should include poison specialists, veterinarians, and registration authorities.

Improving availability

The difficulties experienced in obtaining antidotes for the treatment of poisoned patients vary from country to country. While research in certain areas by industry, and at the international level, could improve the general availability of antidotes, each country will need to identify its own particular problems and take specific action to solve them. A combination of measures will be required, and collaboration will be necessary between the various individuals and organizations involved.

Research and development

Understanding of the metabolism, toxicodynamics, and toxicokinetics of chemicals that cause toxicity in humans can be improved to some extent through animal studies. However, human data are essential and should be obtained from properly conducted clinical studies, ideally using internationally agreed protocols. Better knowledge of the mechanism of action of toxic substances would enable more specific antidotes to be developed.

Appropriate research on antidotes is also essential and should include kinetic, toxicological, and pharmacodynamic studies in both animals and humans. Carefully controlled clinical evaluations of antidotes are often difficult to organize and execute, because of the diversity and relative rarity of poisoning incidents. Proper control of the variables involved is complicated by many factors. For all these reasons, financial support for clinical research should be increased and facilitated, and collaborative studies at both national and international level should be promoted. A concerted effort by the scientific and clinical communities, as well as the pharmaceutical industry, could encourage the development of new antidotes and approval of existing ones for use in humans. This is clearly a long-term process.

Specific studies are also necessary to develop more stable preparations with longer shelf-lives and the ability to withstand a wider range of physical conditions, particularly temperature, light, and humidity. It is important to develop simpler methods of testing the chemical stability and degradation of antidotes under unfavourable physical conditions. Research on more readily usable antidotes is needed, particularly because administration in field conditions by non-medical personnel may be necessary in the event of an emergency. Finally, research could also be directed to the possible inclusion of antidotes with commercial preparations of potentially toxic agents, as has already been done in some countries for paracetamol and methionine.

Action by industry and commerce

The pharmaceutical and chemical industries have an important part to play in the research and development activities referred to above. The pharmaceutical industry could explore ways and means of ensuring the manufacture and distribution of antidotes, including formulations for human and veterinary use which would not normally be made available if commercial criteria alone prevailed. Those industries that use or manufacture toxic chemicals could ensure the availability of, or ready accessibility to, appropriate antidotes at sites used by their workers and at nearby hospitals. This applies also to agricultural activities in which workers may be exposed to both agrochemicals and natural toxins (for example, through the bites of venomous animals) at certain times of the year, such as the planting, crop-spraying, and harvesting seasons. Industrial and commercial enterprises should ensure the proper training of their health personnel in the emergency use of antidotes. Importers and distributors of toxic chemicals should also ensure the availability of specific and effective antidotes for the substances in which they trade.

Action at national level

Poison information centres play a key role in the implementation of a national antidote programme. In general, they are in the unique position of having an overall picture of local poisoning incidents that will enable them to identify the need for specific antidotes in the country as a whole, as well as in particular areas. It is therefore a primary task of these centres to draw attention to the need for making appropriate antidotes available. They should review and evaluate the relevant literature, keep appropriate authorities informed, and facilitate any necessary activities.

Poison information centres should also stimulate the creation of a national network for the supply of antidotes, which will require their close collaboration with the responsible authorities and with hospital pharmacies.

The primary task of authorities at the national level is to ensure that the relevant legislation permits the availability of antidotes, especially those included in the WHO List of Essential Drugs,[1] for purposes of evaluation. Machinery should be set up for the rapid importation, without bureaucratic hindrance, of antidotes for emergency use. Special arrangements may also be needed to permit the controlled clinical use of antidotes that are still under development.

National health authorities should encourage the manufacture and distribution of antidotes not yet available on the local market and could even provide incentives to local pharmaceutical manufacturers, hospital pharmacies, and service laboratories. The export of these antidotes could then also be encouraged. Incentives may be of a financial, fiscal, or similar nature, or provided through the development of human resources and training. National health authorities could also help with, or encourage the organization of, depots for antidotes and systems for the distribution of antidotal agents.

Action at international level

It has been suggested that the establishment of international machinery for the purchase, storage, and distribution of certain antidotes might alleviate the problems of availability in some countries, though it is recognized that this may be difficult to organize and will demand considerable economic resources and political will. If a regional cooperative group could be formed for the supply and storage of antidotes, many of the existing obstacles could be overcome. To this end, regional meetings could be held under the joint auspices of IPCS and WHO Regional Offices to determine a plan of action and to improve cooperation in this area in the various WHO regions.

There is strong support for the suggestion that a list be made of the type and quantities of antidotes immediately available throughout the world. Such a list would allow authorities to locate rarely used antidotes and would also enable large quantities of antidotes to be obtained in the event of a major accident. It would be very difficult, however, to keep the list up to date.

As a result of the IPCS/EC project on antidotes, the WHO List of Essential Drugs has been updated and broadened to include a wider range of antidotes and other substances used in the treatment of poisoning, and it is hoped that this will make national health authorities less reluctant to facilitate the importation of these substances. The preparation of internationally evaluated monographs on each of these substances should also be helpful in this respect. In the same way, the exchanges of

---

[1] *The use of essential drugs. Model List of Essential Drugs (ninth list). Seventh report of the WHO Expert Committee.* Geneva, World Health Organization, 1997 (WHO Technical Report Series, No. 867).

information that take place at international meetings are of great benefit to all those involved.

By making resources and experience available through their development assistance programmes, developed countries could encourage the establishment of storage depots for antidotes in developing countries. With appropriate support, poison information centres in both developed and developing countries could serve as channels for passing on experience, bearing in mind that this is a two-way process. The poison information centres of developing countries could thus gain expertise in the treatment of forms of poisoning that no longer occur commonly in the developed countries, e.g. poisoning by organophosphates.

Where suitable hospital pharmacy facilities exist in developing countries, some antidotes could be prepared locally in cooperation with local poison information centres. Education grants and training courses for pharmaceutical staff in this area would be of value and could be encouraged through international exchange programmes for the development of human resources.

8.
Model formats for collecting, storing, and reporting data

It is an essential function of poison information centres to collect data on chemical substances, on commercial and other products, and on communications (i.e. on enquiries to the centre, requests for information, and reports on poisoning cases). Both the operation of the centre and regular activity reports will be simplified if these data are recorded in standardized formats.

Substance records

To provide advice on management of a patient poisoned by a specific substance, centres must have information on the physical, chemical, and toxicological properties of the substance, its effects on various organ systems and body functions, and diagnostic observations, including results of laboratory tests. The IPCS INTOX Package includes formats for the systematic recording of such information on chemicals, pharmaceuticals, poisonous plants, and poisonous and venomous animals. An example is given in Annex 3.

Product records

A very simple format for recording data on commercial chemical and pharmaceutical products may be adequate, but a more comprehensive format, such as that designed for the IPCS INTOX Package and shown in Annex 4, is recommended.

Communications records

Poison information centres are encouraged to keep systematic records of all their communications, i.e. incoming and outgoing enquiries by telephone, fax, telex, letter, etc., and of personal consultations. Collection of these data is of the utmost importance: they should contain a complete record of any poisoning incident and of any individual poisoned or exposed to poison who has consulted the centre personally or about whom there has been a consultation. The amount of data that should be recorded may vary according to the needs and resources of the centre, as well as the scientific background of the staff in charge of the information service, but records should in any case be as complete as possible. Annex 5 shows the harmonized format developed for use in the IPCS INTOX system. The number of fields used on the record would be decided by the centre concerned, on the basis of its needs and resources, and would depend, among other considerations, on whether data are to be registered on paper or computerized (for which additional items or codes could be included in the form). A harmonized form for case data is valuable in many circumstances but particularly for epidemiological studies and clinical research.

It is not usually possible to complete the clinical case-record fully on a single occasion, and some mechanism should be established for communicating with the responsible treating physician, or even with the patient, in order to collect more data on the evolution and outcome of the case. One such mechanism might be a "follow-up" call or a letter from the centre, asking the physician who treated a poisoned patient to complete the missing information or send a copy of the full record, if this is possible and confidentiality can be guaranteed.

In the case of a regional or global system for the collection of clinical data to permit more extensive epidemiological and clinical research, the model form should be brief and concise. Many of the items that are appropriate to local studies may be irrelevant for global surveys. Further developments in this area are being undertaken by the IPCS.

Annual reports

Centres are encouraged to prepare annual reports of their activities, again using a standardized reporting format. A number of countries have their own annual report formats. In North America, the American Association of Poison Control Centers' Toxic Exposure Surveillance System (TESS) is used. The format prepared by the European Association of Poisons Centres and Clinical Toxicologists (EAPCCT) was subsequently adopted by the European Commission,[1] and consideration is being given to its revision. The proposed format, developed through the IPCS INTOX Project, is given in Annex 6. Further work is being done on this to establish an internationally harmonized format with controlled vocabulary and defined terms.

---

[1] *Official journal of the European Communities*, No. C329/13, 31 December 1990.

9.

Library requirements for poison information centres

Books, journals, and other published literature are indispensable for the work of a poison information centre. There are a number of basic documents that are considered essential for establishing a centre; in addition, specialized literature is needed by staff responsible for patient management or for toxicological analysis. Each centre should have at its disposal documentation that is relevant to the national or regional situation and written, whenever possible, in the local language(s). The main literature requirements include the following:

- indexes, guides, and listings relating to medicines and to agricultural and other chemical products on the local market, plus the local pharmacopoeia
- books or other publications on the animal and plant toxins of the region
- standard textbooks of medicine (general and paediatric), chemistry, pharmacology, and analytical toxicology
- journals of medicine and toxicology
- dictionaries relating to the main areas covered by the documentation in the centre.

It is most important for toxicological data to be kept up to date and maintained in a rational, readily accessible filing system or in a computerized archive. The Microisis System — software developed by the International Development Research Centre of Canada — has proved to be very valuable in this connection, and is generally available through UNESCO or the libraries of local medical schools.

While the volume and complexity of both bibliographical and non-bibliographical data relating to toxicology have greatly increased, the computer can expedite access to them. Many databases may be accessed on-line by telephone, and a growing number of databases are now available on compact disk (CD-ROM) using disk-players that operate in conjunction with relatively inexpensive desk-top computers. The use of computers is thus of enormous value for a centre's information work.

The remainder of this section is devoted to lists of relevant books and journals (most of which are published in English and other major European languages) and to details of other information sources and educational material; these are recommended on the understanding that any centre will have to make its selection in the light of local resources, types of activity, and the principal poisoning problems that occur in the area.

Books

Medical and general toxicology

In English

Baselt RC, Cravey RH. *Disposition of toxic drugs and chemicals in man*, 3rd ed. Chicago, Year Book Medical, 1989.

Dreisbach RH, Robertson WO. *Handbook of poisoning: prevention, diagnosis and treatment*, 12th ed. Los Altos, CA, Appleton & Lange, 1982.

Ellenhorn MJ, Barceloux DG. *Medical toxicology: diagnosis and treatment of human poisoning.* New York, Elsevier, 1988.

Goldfrank LR et al., eds. *Goldfrank's toxicologic emergencies*, 5th ed. Norwalk, CT, Appleton & Lange, 1994.

Gossel TA, Bricker JD. *Principles of clinical toxicology*, 3rd ed. New York, Raven Press, 1984.

Gosselin RE, Smith RP, Hodge HC. *Clinical toxicology of commercial products*, 5th ed. Baltimore, MD, Williams & Wilkins, 1984.

Haddad LM, Winchester JF, eds. *Clinical management of poisoning and drug overdose*, 2nd ed. Philadelphia, Saunders, 1990.

Klaassen CD, ed. *Casarett and Doull's toxicology: the basic science of poisons*, 5th ed. New York, McGraw-Hill, 1996.

Noji EK, Kelen GD, eds. *Manual of toxicologic emergencies.* Chicago, Year Book Medical, 1989.

In French

Baud F, Barriot P, Riou B. *Les antidotes.* Paris, Masson, 1992.

Bismuth C et al. *Toxicologie clinique*, 4th ed. Paris, Flammarion, 1987.

In Italian

Bozza-Marrubini ML, Laurenzi RG, Uccelli P. *Intossicazioni acute: meccanismi, diagnosi e terapia*, 2nd ed. Milan, Organizzazione Editoriale Medico Farmaceutica, 1987.

In Spanish

Astolfi E et al. *Toxicologia de pregrado*, 3rd ed. Buenos Aires, Lopez, 1986.

Dreisbach RH, Robertson WO. *Manual de intoxicaciones: prevención, diagnosis y tratamiento*, 12th ed. Los Altos, CA, Appleton & Lange, 1987.

Fogel de Korc E. *Patología toxicológia.* Oficina del Libro, 1992.

Repetto M. *Toxicológia fundamental.* Madrid, Cientifico Medica, 1987.

In German

Krienke EG et al. *Vergiftungen im Kindesalter*, 2nd ed. Stuttgart, Enke, 1986.

Lindner E. *Toxikologie der Nahrungsmittel.* Thieme, Stuttgart, 1991.

Ludewig R, Lohs KH. *Akute Vergiftungen*, 6th ed. Stuttgart, Fischer, 1981.

Moeschlin S. *Klinik und Therapie der Vergiftungen*, 7th ed. Stuttgart, Thieme, 1986.

Späth G. *Vergiftungen und akute Arzneimittelüberdosierungen*, 2nd ed. Berlin, De Gruyter, 1982.

Velvart J. *Toxikologie der Haushaltprodukte*, 2nd ed. Berne, Huber, 1988.

Wirth W, Gloxhuber C. *Toxikologie*, 4th ed. Stuttgart, Thieme, 1985.

Pharmaceuticals

In English

American Hospital Formulary Service drug information. Bethesda, MD, American Society of Hospital Pharmacists (annual publication).

Briggs GG, Freeman RK, Yaffe JS. *Drugs in pregnancy and lactation: a reference guide to fetal and neonatal risk*, 3rd ed. Baltimore, MD, Williams & Wilkins, 1990.

Davies DM, ed. *Textbook of adverse drug reactions*, 4th ed. Oxford, Oxford University Press, 1991.

Dukes MNG, ed. *Meyler's side effects of drugs: an encyclopedia of adverse reactions and interactions.* 11th ed. Amsterdam, Elsevier, 1989.

Gilman AG et al., eds. *Goodman & Gilman's The pharmacological basis of therapeutics*, 9th ed. New York, Pergamon, 1996.

Hansten PD. *Drug interactions: clinical significance of drug–drug interactions*, 5th ed. Philadelphia, Lea & Febiger, 1985.

Olson KR. *Poisoning and drug overdose*, 2nd ed. Norwalk, CT, Appleton & Lange, 1994.

Physicians' desk reference. Oradell, NJ, Medical Economics (published annually).

Reynolds JEF, ed. *Martindale: the extra pharmacopoeia*, 31st ed. London, Pharmaceutical Press, 1996.

Stockley IH. *Drug interactions*, 3rd ed. Oxford, Blackwell Scientific, 1994.

Occupational and industrial toxicology

In English

Ash M, Ash I. *Thesaurus of chemical products, Vols 1 & 2*, 2nd ed. London, Edward Arnold, 1992.

Budavari S, ed. *Merck index: an encyclopedia of chemicals, drugs and biologicals*, 12th ed. Rahway, NJ, Merck & Co., 1996.

Clayton GD, Clayton FE, eds. *Patty's industrial hygiene and toxicology. Vol. 1, General principles*, 3rd ed. New York, Wiley, 1981.

Clayton GD, Clayton FE, eds. *Patty's industrial hygiene and toxicology, Vols 2A, 2B, 2C, 2D, 2E, 2F*, 4th ed. New York, Wiley, 1993–1994.

Hayes WJ, Laws ER, eds. *Handbook of pesticide toxicology.* San Diego, Academic Press, 1991 (3 volumes).

Lenga RE, Votoupal KL, eds. *The Sigma Aldrich library of chemical safety data.* Milwaukee, Aldrich Chemical Co., 1992.

Proctor NH, Hughes JP, Fischman ML, eds. *Chemical hazards of the workplace*, 3rd ed. Philadelphia, Lippincott, 1991.

Plestina R. *Prevention, diagnosis and treatment of insecticide poisoning.* Geneva, World Health Organization, 1984 (unpublished WHO document WHO/VBC/84.889, obtainable on request from Programme for the Promotion of Chemical Safety, World Health Organization, 1211 Geneva 27, Switzerland).

Rom WN, ed. *Environmental and occupational medicine.* Boston, MA, Little, Brown, 1992.

Sax NI, Lewis RJ, eds. *Dangerous properties of industrial materials*, 8th ed. New York, Van Nostrand Reinhold, 1992.

Sax NI. *Hazardous chemicals desk reference*, 3rd ed. New York, Van Nostrand Reinhold, 1993.

Sax NI. *Rapid guide to hazardous chemicals in the workplace*, 3rd ed. New York, Van Nostrand Reinhold, 1993.

Snyder JR, ed. *Ethel Browning's toxicity and metabolism of industrial solvents.* 2nd ed. Amsterdam, Elsevier, Vol. 1 1987, Vols 2 & 3 1990.

Tomlin C, ed. *The pesticide manual — a world compendium*, 10th ed. Farnham, British Crop Protection Council, 1994.

In French

Encyclopédie Medico-Chirurgicale. *Toxicologie-pathologie professionelle.* Paris, Editions Techniques, 1991.

Lauwerys R. *Toxicologie industrielle et intoxications professionelles*, 3rd ed. Paris, Masson, 1990.

In Spanish

Quer-Brossa S. *Toxicológia industrial*. Barcelona, Salvat Editores, 1983.

In German

Wirkstoffe in Pflanzenschutz und Schädlingsbekämpfungsmitteln, 2nd ed. Frankfurt, Industrieverband Agrar, 1990.

Analytical toxicology

Baselt RC, Cravey RH. *Disposition of toxic drugs and chemicals in man*, 4th ed. Foster City, CA, Chemical Toxicology Institute, 1995.

Curry AS, ed. *Analytical methods in human toxicology, Part 1*. Deerfield Beach, FL, VCH, 1985.

Curry AS, ed. *Analytical methods in human toxicology, Part 2*. Deerfield Beach, FL, VCH, 1986.

Curry AS. *Poison detection in human organs*, 4th ed. Springfield, IL, Charles C. Thomas, 1988.

De Zeeuw RA et al., eds. *Gas-chromatographic retention indices of toxicologically relevant substances on packed or capillary columns with dimethylsilicone stationary phases*, 3rd ed. Deerfield Beach, FL, VCH, 1992.

Eller PM, ed. *NIOSH manual of analytical methods, Vol. 1*, 3rd ed. Cincinnati, OH, National Institute of Occupational Safety and Health, 1984.

Environmental health criteria. Geneva, World Health Organization (series).

Feigl F. *Spot tests in organic analysis*, 7th ed. Amsterdam, Elsevier, 1966.

Flanagan RJ et al. *Basic analytical toxicology*. Geneva, World Health Organization, 1995.

Moffat AC et al., eds. *Clarke's isolation and identification of drugs in pharmaceuticals, body fluids, and post-mortem material*, 2nd ed. London, Pharmaceutical Press, 1986.

Stewart CP, Stolman A. *Toxicology: mechanism and analytical methods, Vol. 1*. New York and London, Academic Press, 1960.

Stewart CP, Stolman A. *Toxicology: mechanism and analytical methods, Vol 2*. New York and London, Academic Press, 1961.

Sunshine I. *Methodology for analytical toxicology*. Cleveland, OH, Chemical Rubber Company Press, 1975.

United Nations Division of Narcotic Drugs. *Recommended methods for testing: manuals for use by national narcotics laboratories*. New York, United Nations, 1984–1989.[1]

World Health Organization/Food and Agriculture Organization. *Data sheets on pesticides* (unpublished WHO documents, available on request from Programme for the Promotion of Chemical Safety, World Health Organization, 1211 Geneva 27, Switzerland).

Natural poisons

Books on natural poisons should be selected according to the real incidence of risks of poisoning by animals or plants in the geographical area concerned. Illustrated guides,

---

[1] Separate publications for testing different substances.

with drawings, photographs, or even specimens, are very useful for the identification of local plants and animals (fungi, snakes, spiders, scorpions, insects, marine animals, etc.). Most of the valuable literature will therefore come from the geographical area itself, but certain books can be recommended, since natural toxins are distributed worldwide.

Bresinsky A, Besl H. *A colour atlas of poisonous fungi: a handbook for pharmacists, doctors and biologists.* London, Wolfe, 1990.

Frohne D, Pfändner HJ. *A colour atlas of poisonous plants: a handbook for pharmacists, doctors, toxicologists, and biologists.* London, Wolfe, 1984.

Halstead BW. *Poisonous and venomous marine animals of the world*, 2nd ed. Princeton, NJ, Darwin Press, 1988.

Lampe KF, McCann MA. *American Medical Association handbook of poisonous and injurious plants.* Chicago, American Medical Association, 1985.

Lincott G, Mitchel DH. *Toxic and hallucinogenic mushroom poisoning.* New York, Van Nostrand Reinhold, 1977.

Specialized toxicology

Publications specializing in toxicology of the eye, central nervous system, heart, lung, kidney, liver, and skin, as well as books on toxins and cancer, on effects of drugs in pregnancy and lactation, and on drugs of abuse, may be required whenever information is needed on specific target organs or systems. Examples include the following:

Barken RM. Rosen P, eds. *Emergency paediatrics: a guide for emergency and urgent care*, 4th ed. St Louis, MO, CV Mosby, 1993.

Briggs GG, Freeman RK, Yaffe SJ. *Drugs in pregnancy and lactation: a reference guide to fetal and neonatal risk*, 4th ed. Baltimore, MD, Williams & Wilkins, 1994.

Descotes J. *Immunotoxicology of drugs and chemicals*, 2nd ed. Amsterdam, Elsevier, 1988.

Fisher AA. *Contact dermatitis*, 3rd ed. Philadelphia, Lea & Febiger, 1986.

Grant WM, Schuman JS. *Toxicology of the eye*, 4th ed. Springfield, IL, Charles C. Thomas, 1993.

Books dealing with veterinary toxicology may be helpful in some cases. Examples include the following:

In English

Bartik M, Piskac A. *Veterinary toxicology.* New York, Elsevier, 1981.

Booth NH, McDonald LE. *Veterinary pharmacology and therapeutics*, 6th ed. Ames, IA, Iowa State University Press, 1988.

Garner RJ et al. *Veterinary toxicology*, 3rd ed. London, Balliere Tindall, 1988.

Howard J. *Current veterinary therapy: food animal practice.* Philadelphia, Saunders, 1986.

Kirk RW. *Current veterinary therapy: small animal practice.* Philadelphia, Saunders/Harcourt-Brace Jovanovich, 1989.

Osweiler GD et al. *Clinical and diagnostic veterinary toxicology*, 3rd ed. Dubuque, IA, Kendall/Hunt, 1985.

Robinson NE. *Current therapy in equine medicine*, 2nd ed. Phildelphia, Saunders, 1987.

In German

Hapke HJ. *Toxikologie für Veterinärmediziner.* Stuttgart, Ferdinand Enke, 1988.

Books on eco-toxicology and environmental toxicology are also important, as poison information centres are frequently involved in, or consulted about, the management and assessment of environmental problems and their effects on health.

Bearing in mind that the information requested from a centre can sometimes involve highly specialized branches of medicine, it is recommended that the centre — or other readily accessible libraries — have well known, up-to-data textbooks on paediatrics, nephrology, hepatology, lung diseases, gastroenterology, cardiology, ophthalmology, gynaecology and obstetrics, dermatology, psychiatry, etc.

Journals

A list of some of the numerous periodicals that deal essentially with toxicology or closely related areas is given below. It should be noted that, in many countries, there are local journals on toxicology, usually published by national scientific associations. It is recommended that any poison information centres should also have access to journals devoted to more general clinical, industrial, chemical, and ecological topics.

In English

Adverse drug reactions and toxicological reviews. Published by Oxford University Press, Oxford, England.
American journal of industrial medicine. Published by Wiley, New York, NY, USA.
Annals of occupational hygiene. Published by Pergamon, Elmsford, NY, USA.
Archives of environmental contamination and toxicology. Published by Springer Verlag, New York, USA.
Archives of environmental health. Published by Heldref (Helen Dwight Reid Educational Foundation), Washington, DC, USA.
Archives of toxicology. Published by Springer Verlag, Berlin, USA.
Biochemical pharmacology. Published by Pergamon, Elmsford, NY, USA.
British journal of industrial medicine. Published by British Medical Association, London, England.
Drug safety (formerly *Medical toxicology*). Published by ADIS Press, Auckland, New Zealand.
EHP (Environmental health perspectives). Published by US Department of Health and Human Services, National Institute of Environmental Health Sciences, Research Triangle Park, NC, USA.
Human and experimental toxicology. Published by Macmillan, Basingstoke, England.
Journal of the American Industrial Hygiene Association. Published by American Industrial Hygiene Association, Akron, OH, USA.
Journal of toxicology — clinical toxicology. Published by Marcel Dekker Inc., New York, NY, USA.
Neurotoxicology. Published by Raven Press, New York, USA.
Pharmacology and toxicology. Published by Munksgaard, Copenhagen, Denmark.
Scandinavian journal of work, environment and health. Published by Finnish Institute of Occupational Health, Helsinki, Finland.
Toxicology. Published by Elsevier, Limerick, Ireland.
Toxicology and applied pharmacology. Published by Academic Press, San Diego, CA, USA.
Toxicology letters. Published by Elsevier, Amsterdam, Netherlands.
Toxicon. Published by Pergamon, Elmsford, NY, USA.

Veterinary and human toxicology. Published by Comparative Toxicology Laboratories, Manhattan, KS, USA.

In French

Archives belges de médecine sociale et d'hygiène (formerly *Archives belges de médecine sociale, hygiène, médecine du travail et médecine légale*). Published by Archives belges de médecine sociale et d'hygiène, Brussels, Belgium.
Archives des maladies professionnelles de médecine du travail et de sécurité sociale. Published by Masson, Paris, France.
Thérapie. Published by Doin, Paris, France.

In Italian

Medicina del lavoro. Published by Istituti Clinici di Perfezionamento, Milan, Italy.

In Spanish

Toxicología. Published by Sociedad Uruguaya de Toxicología y Ecotoxicología del Uruguay, Montevideo, Uruguay.

Access to other medical journals that may contain reports of relevance to the work of the centre is recommended, notably those dealing with emergency medicine, epidemiology, intensive care, occupational medicine, pharmacology and adverse drug reactions, clinical medicine, paediatrics, public health, and psychiatry. Journals and newsletters published by agencies dealing with accident prevention or associations that undertake research in this area may also be useful.

Current awareness publications, abstracts, and bibliographical indexes are useful for updating information. Although they are expensive, they are usually available at teaching hospitals and in university libraries. They include:

- *Medline*
- *Toxline*
- *Reactions*
- *Current contents*
- *Toxicology abstracts*
- *Excerpta medica*
- *Index medicus*

Publications of international organizations

The Environmental Health Criteria series published by WHO provides valuable data on priority chemicals (see Annex 7).

Poison information centres may also derive useful information from certain publications produced by the Food and Agriculture Organization of the United Nations, the International Labour Organisation, the International Register of Potentially Toxic Chemicals, and the United Nations Environment Programme. Centres should ask the local representatives or national correspondents of these agencies for lists of their publications.

Monographs from the International Agency for Research on Cancer on the evaluation of the carcinogenic risk of chemicals to humans provide reliable, up-to-date information on a large number of chemicals (contact IARC, 158 Cours Albert-Thomas, 69372 Lyon Cedex 08, France).

Computerized databases

Computerized databases provide easy, on-line access to a wide range of useful information, but may be expensive to maintain. Some databases (e.g. Dialog, CIS, Medline, Toxline) have already been adopted by the more experienced poison information centres, but the more specific ones should be carefully chosen according to local needs and resources. A comprehensive list of databases can be provided on request from IPCS, World Health Organization, 1211 Geneva 27, Switzerland.

Educational material

Educational material is sometimes produced by government agencies, nongovernmental organizations, manufacturers' associations, scientific societies, accident prevention agencies, and other institutions interested in the prevention and correct management of poisoning. Such material can also be produced by the staff of poison information centres for the training of professional health care workers and others or for the information of the community.

For example, the library at a poison information centre may have, for distribution, a government-produced poster on the safe use of pesticides; it may design and print a leaflet on the safe storage of medicines at home; it may distribute a booklet on the recognition of poisonous fungi; or it may develop, for distribution to clinicians, highly specialized protocols for the treatment of the most common types of poisoning.

Posters, booklets, leaflets, bulletins, video cassettes, or audiovisual displays relevant to the local situation should also be available at the centre's library.

Annexes

Annex I
Summary description of the IPCS INTOX Package[1]

The essential component of the IPCS INTOX Package is a computer software system for data management of poisons information. Although it is aimed primarily at the needs of the information services of poison centres in developing countries, the Package is also very suitable for use in developed countries with well established centres. It is designed to be operated in English, French, and Spanish, but versions for other languages can easily be developed. Moreover, the system can be operated on a stand-alone personal computer, a network of computers within a single centre, a network of centres within a country, and internationally. The software system is delivered with a CD-ROM containing Poisons Information Monographs and various other publications designed to be useful to poison centres, as well as the electronic versions of the system documentation. The software and the CD-ROM constitute the IPCS INTOX Package. The Package is the result of a continuing IPCS INTOX project carried out under the aegis of IPCS.

Definitions

The following paragraphs provide definitions of a number of terms employed in the IPCS INTOX Package:

- An "entity" is something that can enter the body of a human or animal; it is either a substance or a product, or a class of substances or of products. Any chemical to which an individual is exposed may be termed an entity. Substances and products are classified either by their scientific group (or family for a plant or animal) or by their function.

- A "substance" is a chemical or pharmaceutical of natural or synthetic origin, or produced by the biological processes of an organism such as a poisonous plant or a poisonous or venomous animal.

- A "product" is a substance or preparation (i.e. mixture of substances) placed on the market, normally with a unique designation or brand name.

- An "agent" is a specific instance of an entity and is the linkage between the substance, product components of the Package, and the communications component. The agent is the poison or supposed toxic substance or class thereof to which a communication refers.

- A "communication" is any interaction between a poison information centre and its interlocutors or clients. It usually takes the form of a telephone call, incoming or outgoing, but may also be a fax, letter, telex, or face-to-face contact.

---

[1] Developed by IPCS in association with the Canadian Centre for Occupational Health and Safety (CCOHS) and the Centre de Toxicologie du Québec (CTQ), with financial assistance from the International Development Research Centre (IDRC) of Canada and Member States of WHO. Further information about the Package and its availability can be obtained from the Director, IPCS, World Health Organization, 1211 Geneva 27, Switzerland.

- An "interlocutor" or "client" is the individual or institution with whom the poison information centre is communicating.

- An "authority list" is a series of controlled or harmonized terms used for data entry into, and data retrieval from, the IPCS INTOX Package. In some cases the authority list is fixed by the project and cannot be altered, e.g. Sex — Male, Female, Unknown. In some cases there is a proposed list of terms to which a centre can add its own terms, but from which it cannot delete existing terms; in other cases the centre is free to develop its own authority list.

Databases

The IPCS INTOX system maintains two interrelated databases, each of which uses standardized formats — the "entity" database and the "communications" database. The entity database contains details of substances and commercial and other products (including their synonyms). There are standardized formats for information on substances — chemicals and pharmaceuticals, plus the toxic substances contained in poisonous plants and in poisonous and venomous animals — and on commercial and other products that contain substances. Classes of substances and of products, classified either by scientific group or by function, are also part of the entity database and have their own standardized formats.

The communications database contains records of the interactions between the poison information centre and its interlocutors or clients. The names and synonyms of all the entities, including classes, held by the system constitute the authority list for inclusion in the communications records of the names of agents. The use of entity names as agent names forms the link between the two databases.

As far as possible data are entered using controlled or harmonized terms chosen from authority lists. These authority lists are either generated globally by the project through consensus, or locally by the centre itself. This comprehensive use of controlled vocabularies is a prerequisite for the storage of high-quality information which can be reliably retrieved and analysed. The use of controlled terms facilitates data entry and retrieval, as well as permitting the user to "navigate" the database.

Substance records

The format on substances enables a "substance record" to be created, containing data on the physico-chemical and toxicological properties of a substance, on the medical features of the effects produced by various routes of exposure to the substance, on management of patients, and on supporting laboratory investigations. Most of the data on substances are globally valid and may be found in the scientific literature or are generated as a result of the overall work of IPCS on risk assessment of chemicals. In order to assist poison information centres, particularly new centres, to develop their own databases on substances, a series of Poisons Information Monographs (PIMs) is being prepared on priority substances selected because of their importance as causes of poisoning or as subjects of enquiries to poison information centres, particularly in developing countries. The PIMs are issued as IPCS documents and are also made available to the IPCS INTOX project on a CD-ROM which is produced for the IPCS by the Canadian Centre for Occupational Health and Safety. PIMs can be imported from the CD-ROM into the IPCS INTOX database on the computer at the centre.

While the formats of the PIMs are the same as those for the substance records in the IPCS INTOX database, it is not necessary to have a completed PIM in order to have a substance record. The only essential part of the substance record for the operation of the

IPCS INTOX Package is the substance name, which is important, since it means that the database at a poison information centre using the IPCS INTOX Package is not limited only to information for which there is a PIM. Each centre may build up its own database containing substances of relevance to its own situation, adding the essential data from the PIMs as they become available or as they are subsequently revised or updated.

The format for PIMs and substance records is given in Annex 3. The formats for chemicals, pharmaceuticals, poisonous plants, and poisonous and venomous animals are, with some small modifications to the contents, more or less identical. Guidelines are provided in the User's Manual for the IPCS INTOX Package on preparing PIMs and substance records.

Product records

The format on commercial products enables a product record to be created containing data on the manufacturer, distributor, or importer of a commercial product, on how the product is presented (packaging), on its characteristics (form and physico-chemical properties), and composition, on relevant toxicological data, and on patient management.

The format is adapted for both commercial products containing chemicals and commercial preparations of pharmaceuticals. It remains to be seen in practice whether it is fully adaptable to non-commercial products, such as traditional medicines and locally fabricated products of variable composition found in bazaars and markets. The format for the product record is given in Annex 4. Guidelines on completing a product record are provided in the User's Manual for the IPCS INTOX Package.

Classes of substances

In a case of poisoning it is not always possible to identify the specific substance(s) or product(s) involved, but rather a class or group — an organophosphate, a benzodiazepine, a pesticide, a rat-killer, a dish-washing liquid, a solvent, a painkiller, etc. Any such class or group could be the name of the agent (poison) given by an enquirer (interlocutor) in a call (communication) to a poison information centre. The IPCS INTOX Package enables class records to be created so that classes and groups and their synonyms may be included in the entity database. The "Category of Use" or function field in the product record and the "Group" or "Family" fields in the substance record are made from the list of classes and their synonyms. Class structures may be complex, with a substance or product being a member of more than one class. Further-more, a class record may pertain to more than one type of substance or product. The IPCS INTOX Package enables one class record to be linked to another. Each class record may have zero or any number of links created in it.

Communications record

The format on communications enables a poison information centre to record and retrieve information on any incoming or outgoing telephone call, fax, telex, letter or face-to-face contact: the person or institution (interlocutor) with whom the centre is interacting; an incident (single or multiple), and the type, location, and circumstances involved; a patient or patients and various related details; and various agent(s)/route(s). One contact with the poison information centre defines one communication which may, for example, involve several different types of enquiry. One or more contact or communication dealing with the same incident/patient combination defines the basis of a case. The cumulative data at a poison information centre on a case may or may not constitute a full clinical case record. International work being undertaken in the context of the IPCS to define and harmonize medical features of effects of poisoning and their severity, as well as descriptions of treatment procedures, is at a preliminary stage and it will be a number of years before it is possible to consider establishing a fully harmonized hospital case data record for global use. Likewise, much work remains to be done on harmonizing the description of laboratory investigations associated with diagnosis, prognosis, and management of poisoned patients. The available version of the IPCS INTOX Package incorporates the current consensus on clinical features and severity grading. The format for recording a communication is given in Annex 5. Guidelines on recording a communication are available in the User's Manual for the IPCS INTOX Package.

Other types of record

A number of auxiliary databases are also provided with the IPCS INTOX Package. These enable centres to record the names, addresses, and functions of various individuals and medical and other institutions with which the poison information centre is in frequent contact.

Interaction with other packages

It is intended that future versions of the IPCS INTOX Package will be able to interface with other packages, such as plant and tablet identification packages, as well as packages for performing mathematical computations, e.g. transforming one set of units into another (pounds to kilograms, feet to metres, etc.).

Hardware and software specifications

The IPCS INTOX software system will operate on a personal computer with the Microsoft Windows[1] operating system (version 3.1 or later); MS-DOS 5.0 or later is also necessary. The recommended hardware arrangement is an 80486 processor, running at a minimum of 33 MHz, 8 Mb of RAM, a colour display capable of handling SVGA resolution (800 × 600), a 3.5" floppy disk drive, a CD-ROM drive, and a mouse. The required capacity of the hard disk will depend on the amount of information that will be collected by the centre: 120 Mb should be considered the absolute minimum. The CD-ROM player is required to access the database of PIMs and other material. A printer of any type that is compatible with the system described is also recommended, depending on the quality of the output required by the centre. The preferred informatics specifications for the IPCS INTOX Package are given in the User's Manual.

With future versions of the IPCS INTOX Package it will be possible to incorporate colour pictures and drawings, which are of particular value in the identification of poisonous plants and poisonous and venomous animals. This capability may also be useful in illustrating clinical features such as rashes and bites, as well as packaging materials and characteristics of commercial products.

Support to users of the IPCS INTOX Package

The IPCS INTOX system development staff and other informatics experts in various parts of the world are accessible by fax, electronic mail, and telephone. In addition, the

---

[1] Microsoft is a registered trademark and Windows is a trademark of the Microsoft Corporation.

IPCS INTOX project operates a twinning arrangement among poison centres that wish to participate in such an arrangement, so that they can give each other mutual support, and "discussions" between members of the project can take place on the Internet network using electronic mail.

Annex 2
Classified lists of antidotes and other agents

Group 1   List of antidotes
Group 2   Agents used to prevent the absorption of poisons, to enhance their elimination, or to treat symptomatically their effects on body functions
Group 3   Other useful therapeutic agents for the treatment of poisoning
Group 4   List of antidotes and related agents considered obsolete

The antidotes listed in Groups 1 and 2 are considered useful in the treatment of acute human poisoning, and their availability in terms of urgency of use may be classified as follows:

A   Required to be immediately available (within 30 minutes).
B   Required to be available within 2 hours.
C   Required to be available within 6 hours.

Their effectiveness in practice may be classified as follows:

1   Effectiveness well documented, e.g. reduction of lethality in animal experiments and reduction of lethality or of severe complications in human poisoning.
2   Widely used but not yet universally accepted as effective, owing to lack of research data, and requiring further investigation concerning effectiveness or indications for use.
3   Questionable usefulness; as many data as possible regarding effectiveness should be collected.

The classification in terms of urgency of availability (A, B, C) or proven effectiveness (1, 2, 3) is given next to the main indication for the antidote. The classification is also given in the right-hand column of the Group 1 list when an antidote has other possible applications. If there is doubt as to the classification of an antidote, the lower score is always given, e.g. B2 instead of A1.

Group 1. Antidotes

Antidote	Main indication or pathological condition	Other possible applications
acetylcysteine	paracetamol (B1)	
N-acetyl penicillamine	mercury (inorganic and vapour) (C3)	
amyl nitrite	cyanide (A2)	
atropine[a,b]	organophosphorus compounds and carbamates (A1)	
benzylpenicillin[a]	amanitins (B3)	
β-blockers (β$_1$ and β$_2$, preferably short-acting)	β-adrenergic agonists (A1)	theophylline (B1)
calcium gluconate or other soluble calcium salts[a]	HF, fluorides, oxalates (A1)	calcium antagonists (B3)
dantrolene	drug-induced hyperthermia (A2)	malignant neuroleptic syndrome (A2)
deferoxamine[a,b]	iron (B1)	aluminium (C2)
diazepam[a]	organophosphates (A2)	chloroquine (A2)
dicobalt edetate	cyanide (A1)	
digoxin-specific antibodies (Fab fragments)	digoxin/digitoxin, other digitalis glycosides (A1)	
dimercaprol[a,b]	arsenic (B3)	gold (C3), mercury (inorganic) (C3)
4-dimethylaminophenol (4-DMAP)	cyanide (A1)	
edetate calcium disodium (CaNa$_2$-EDTA)	lead (C2)	
ethanol	methanol, ethylene glycol (A1)	
flumazenil	benzodiazepines (B1)	
folinic acid	folinic acid antagonists (B1)	methanol (B3)
glucagon	β-blockers (A1)	
glucose (hypertonic)	insulin (A1)	
hydroxocobalamin[a]	cyanide (A1)	
isoprenaline[a]	β-blockers (A1)	
methionine[a,b]	paracetamol (B1)	
4-methylpyrazole[c]	ethylene glycol (A1)	methanol, coprin, disulfiram (B2)
methylthioninium chloride (methylene blue)[a,b]	methaemoglobinaemia (A1)	
naloxone[a]	opiates (A1)	
neostigmine[a]	neuromuscular block (curare type), peripheral anticholinergic efects (B2)	
obidoxime	organophosphorus insecticides (B2)	
oxygen[a]	cyanide, carbon monoxide, hydrogen sulfide (A1)	
oxygen, hyperbaric	carbon monoxide (C2)	cyanide, hydrogen sulfide, carbon tetrachloride

Antidote	Main indication or pathological condition	Other possible applications
penicillamine[a,b]	copper (Wilson disease) (C1)	lead, mercury (inorganic) (C2)
pentetic acid (DTPA)	cobalt (C3)	radioactive metals
phentolamine	α-adrenergic poisoning (A1)	
physostigmine	central anticholinergic syndrome from atropine and derivatives (A1)	central anticholinergic syndrome from other drugs
phytomenadione (vitamin K$_1$)[a]	coumarin derivatives (C1)	
potassium ferric hexacyanoferrate (Prussian blue C177520)[a,b]	thallium (B2)	
pralidoxime	organophosphorus compounds	
prenalterol	β-blockers (A1)	
propranolol (see β-blockers)		
protamine sulfate[a]	heparin (A1)	
pyridoxine[a]	isoniazid, hydrazines (A2)	ethylene glycol (C3), gyrometrine (B2)
silibinin	amanitin (B2)	
sodium nitrite[a,b]	cyanide (A1)	
sodium nitroprusside[a]	ergotism (A1)	
sodium thiosulfate[a,b]	cyanide (A1)	bromate, chlorate, iodate
succimer (DMSA)	antimony, arsenic, bismuth, cadmium, cobalt, copper, gold, lead, mercury (organic and inorganic) (B2)	mercury (elemental), platinum, silver (C3)
trientine (triethylene tetramine)	copper (Wilson disease) (C2)	
unithiol (DMPS)	cobalt, gold, lead, mercury (inorganic), nickel (C2)	cadmium, mercury (organic) (C3)

[a] Listed in the WHO Model List of Essential Drugs (see: *The use of essential drugs. Model List of Essential Drugs (ninth list). Seventh report of the WHO Expert Committee.* Geneva, World Health Organization, 1997 (WHO Technical Report Series, No. 867)).

[b] Evaluated or under evaluation by group of experts on behalf of IPCS/CEC.

[c] Available only in France.

Group 2. Agents used to prevent the absorption of poisons, to enhance their elimination, or to treat symptomatically their effects on body functions

Emetics
   apomorphine
   ipecacuanha

Cathartics and solutions for whole gut lavage
   magnesium citrate/sulfate/hydroxide (B3)
   mannitol/sorbitol/lactulose (B3)
   sodium sulfate/phosphate/bicarbonate (B3)
   polyethylene glycol electrolyte lavage solution (B2)

Agents to alkalinize urine or blood
    sodium bicarbonate (A1)

Agents to prevent absorption of toxic substances in the gastrointestinal tract
activated charcoal (A1)	— for adsorbable poisons
starch (A3)	— for iodine

Agents to prevent skin absorption and/or damage
calcium gluconate gel (A1)	— for hydrofluoric acid
polyethylene glycol (Macrogol 400)	— for phenol

Anti-foaming agent
dimethicone[a]	— for soaps, shampoos

Group 3. Other therapeutic agents useful for the treatment of poisoning

Listed below are certain therapeutic agents that are not antidotes according to the accepted definition; however, because of their established value and sometimes specific role in the management of poisoning, they border on the concept of antidotes. In practice, these agents are used frequently in cases of poisoning and in other medical circumstances. Most of them are considered to be essential drugs and should therefore be available for immediate use.

Agent	Indications/symptoms arising from poisoning
benztropine	dystonia
chlorpromazine	psychotic states with severe agitation
corticosteroids	acute allergic reactions, laryngeal oedema (systemic/topical) bronchoconstriction, mucosal oedema (inhaled)
diazepam	convulsions, excitation, anxiety, muscular hypertonia
diphenhydramine	dystonia
dobutamine	myocardial depression
dopamine	myocardial depression, vascular relaxation
epinephrine (adrenaline)	anaphylactic shock, cardiac arrest
furosemide	fluid retention, left ventricular failure
glucose	hypoglycaemia
haloperidol	hallucinatory and psychotic states
heparin	hypercoagulability states
magnesium sulfate	cardiac arrhythmias
mannitol	cerebral oedema, fluid retention
oxygen	hypoxia
pancuronium	muscular rigidity, convulsions
promethazine	allergic reactions
salbutamol	bronchoconstriction (systemic/inhaled)
sodium bicarbonate	acidosis, some cardiac disturbances

---

[a] To be evaluated.

Group 4. List of antidotes and related agents now considered obsolete

Antidote	Indicated for
acetazolamide	modification of urinary pH
ascorbic acid	methaemoglobinaemia
aurintricarboxylic acid (ATA)	beryllium
β-aminopropionitrile	caustics
castor oil	as cathartic
copper sulfate	as emetic
cyclophosphamide	gold-paraquat
cysteamine	paracetamol
diethyldithiocarbamate	thallium
fructose	ethanol
guanidine precursors	botulism
levallorphan	opiates
nalorphine	opiates
potassium permanganate	fluorides
sodium chloride	as emetic
sodium salicylate	beryllium
strychnine	central nervous system depressants
sulfadimidine	amanitine
tannins	alkaloids
thioctic acid	amanitine
tocopherol (vitamin E)	paraquat
tolonium chloride	methaemoglobinaemia
universal antidote	ingested poisons

Annex 3
Example of a substance record: chemical

1. **Name**
    1.1   Substance
    1.2   Group
    1.3   Synonyms
    1.4   Identification numbers
        1.4.1   Chemical Abstracts Service (CAS)
        1.4.2   Other numbers
    1.5   Main brand names/main trade names
    1.6   Main manufacturers and/or importers

2. **Summary**
    2.1   Main risks and target organs
    2.2   Summary of clinical effects
    2.3   Diagnosis
    2.4   First-aid measures and management principles

3. **Physico-chemical properties**
    3.1   Origin of the substance
    3.2   Chemical structure
    3.3   Physical properties
    3.4   Other characteristics

4. **Uses/high-risk circumstances of poisoning**
    4.1   Uses
    4.2   High-risk circumstance of poisoning
    4.3   Occupationally exposed populations

5. **Routes of entry**
    5.1   Oral
    5.2   Inhalation
    5.3   Dermal
    5.4   Eye
    5.5   Parenteral
    5.6   Others

6. **Kinetics**
    6.1   Absorption by route of exposure
    6.2   Distribution by route of exposure
    6.3   Biological half-life by route of exposure
    6.4   Metabolism
    6.5   Elimination by route of exposure

7. **Toxicology**
   7.1 Mode of action
   7.2 Toxicity
    7.2.1 Human data
     7.2.1.1 Adults
     7.2.1.2 Children
    7.2.2 Relevant animal data
    7.2.3 Relevant *in-vitro* data
    7.2.4 Workplace standards
    7.2.5 Acceptable daily intake (ADI) and other guideline levels
   7.3 Carcinogenicity
   7.4 Teratogenicity
   7.5 Mutagenicity
   7.6 Interactions

8. **Toxicological analyses and biomedical investigations**
   8.1 Material sampling plan
    8.1.1 Sampling and specimen collection
     8.1.1.1 Toxicological analyses
     8.1.1.2 Biomedical analyses
     8.1.1.3 Arterial blood-gas analyses
     8.1.1.4 Haematological analyses
     8.1.1.5 Other (unspecified) analyses
    8.1.2 Storage of laboratory samples and specimens
     8.1.2.1 Toxicological analyses
     8.1.2.2 Biomedical analyses
     8.1.2.3 Arterial blood-gas analyses
     8.1.2.4 Haematological analyses
     8.1.2.5 Other (unspecified) analyses
    8.1.3 Transport of laboratory samples and specimens
     8.1.3.1 Toxicological analyses
     8.1.3.2 Biomedical analyses
     8.1.3.3 Arterial blood-gas analyses
     8.1.3.4 Haematological analyses
     8.1.3.5 Other (unspecified) analyses
   8.2 Toxicological analyses and their interpretation
    8.2.1 Tests on toxic ingredient(s) of material
     8.2.1.1 Simple qualitative test(s)
     8.2.1.2 Advanced qualitative confirmation test(s)
     8.2.1.3 Simple quantitative method(s)
     8.2.1.4 Advanced quantitative method(s)
    8.2.2 Tests for biological specimens
     8.2.2.1 Simple qualitative test(s)
     8.2.2.2 Advanced qualitative confirmation test(s)
     8.2.2.3 Simple quantitative method(s)
     8.2.2.4 Advanced quantitative method(s)
     8.2.2.5 Other dedicated method(s)
    8.2.3 Interpretation of toxicological analyses
   8.3 Biomedical investigations and their interpretation
    8.3.1 Biochemical analyses
     8.3.1.1 Blood, plasma or serum:

          — basic analyses
          — dedicated analyses
          — optional analyses
    8.3.1.2 Urine:
          — basic analyses
          — dedicated analyses
          — optional analyses
    8.3.1.3 Other fluids
  8.3.2 Arterial blood-gas analyses
  8.3.3 Haematological analyses:
          — basic analyses
          — dedicated analyses
          — optional analyses
  8.3.4 Interpretation of biomedical investigations
8.4 Other biomedical (diagnostic) investigations and their interpretation
8.5 Overall interpretation of all toxicological analyses and biomedical investigations
8.6 References

9. **Clinical effects**
  9.1 Acute poisoning
    9.1.1 Ingestion
    9.1.2 Inhalation
    9.1.3 Skin exposure
    9.1.4 Eye contact
    9.1.5 Parenteral exposure
    9.1.6 Others
  9.2 Chronic poisoning
    9.2.1 Ingestion
    9.2.2 Inhalation
    9.2.3 Skin exposure
    9.2.4 Eye contact
    9.2.5 Parenteral exposure
    9.2.6 Others
  9.3 Course, prognosis, cause of death
  9.4 Systematic description of clinical effects
    9.4.1 Cardiovascular
    9.4.2 Respiratory
    9.4.3 Neurological
      9.4.3.1 Central nervous system
      9.4.3.2 Peripheral nervous system
      9.4.3.3 Autonomic nervous system
      9.4.3.4 Skeletal and smooth muscle
    9.4.4 Gastrointestinal
    9.4.5 Hepatic
    9.4.6 Urinary
      9.4.6.1 Renal
      9.4.6.2 Others
    9.4.7 Endocrine and reproductive systems
    9.4.8 Dermatological
    9.4.9 Eyes, ears, nose, throat: local effects

9.4.10 Haematological

9.4.11 Immunological

9.4.12 Metabolic

9.4.12.1 Acid–base disturbances

9.4.12.2 Fluid and electrolyte disturbances

9.4.12.3 Others

9.4.13 Allergic reactions

9.4.14 Other clinical effects

9.4.15 Special risks: pregnancy, breast-feeding, enzyme deficiencies

9.5 Others

10. **Management**

10.1 General principles

10.2 Relevant laboratory analyses and other investigations

10.2.1 Sample collection

10.2.2 Biomedical analyses

10.2.3 Toxicological analyses

10.2.4 Other investigations

10.3 Life-supportive procedures and symptomatic treatment

10.4 Decontamination

10.5 Elimination

10.6 Antidote treatment

10.6.1 Adults

10.6.2 Children

10.7 Management discussion: alternatives, controversies, and research needs

11. **Illustrative cases**

11.1 Case reports from literature

11.2 Internally extracted data on cases (from the writer of the monograph)

11.3 Internal cases (added by the poison centre using monograph)

12. **Additional information**

12.1 Availability of antidotes and sera

12.2 Specific preventive measures

12.3 Other

13. **References**

14. **Author(s), reviewer(s), date (including each update), complete addresses**

Annex 4
INTOX product record

INTOX PRODUCT RECORD

CONFIDENTIAL

1. *IDENTITY*

1.1 Product name		

1.2 Other name(s)	1.3 Function

1.4 Legal category

1.5 Manufacturer

Name	Address	Telephone
		Fax/Telex

1.6 Distributor

Name	Address	Telephone
		Fax/Telex

1.7 Importer

Name	Address	Telephone
		Fax/Telex

1.8 Contact point

1.9 Country of origin

2. *PRESENTATION/PACK*

2.1 State/Form

2.2 Description

3. *COMPOSITION*

3.1 Major constituents	3.2 Other constituents

4. *CHARACTERISTICS*

4.1 Colour	4.8 Flashpoint
4.2 Odour	4.9 Stability
4.3 pH 4.3.1 As supplied: 4.3.2 When used:	4.10 Reactivity
4.4 Viscosity	4.11 Hazardous combustion
4.5 Volatility	4.12 Hazardous polymerization
4.6 Solubility	4.13 Hazardous degradation products
4.7 Flammability	4.14 Shelf-life
	4.15 Corrosivity

5. MANDATORY REQUIREMENTS RELATING TO SAFETY

5.1 Requirements

5.2 Comments

6. WARNING FLAG

7. ENDORSEMENT

7.1 Company

7.2 Date of first marketing of the product	7.3 Product replaces

8. TOXICOLOGY DATA

(Animal, human, other)

9. KINETICS

10. CLINICAL EFFECTS

10.1 Clinical features

10.2 Comments

11. MANAGEMENT

12. ILLUSTRATIVE CASES

Annex 5
INTOX communication record
and miniform

INTOX-COMMUNICATION RECORD	Page 1 of 4		1.1 No	☐☐☐☐☐☐

Version 3

1. COMMUNICATION		1.2 Date dd/mm/yy ☐☐ ☐☐ ☐☐	1.3 Time ☐ : ☐

1.4 Officer

1.1 Topic

1.5 Method

	Incoming	Outgoing
Phone call	☐	☐
Letter	☐	☐
Fax/Telex	☐	☐
Questionnaire	☐	☐

☐ Personal contact

☐ Other

1.6 Reasons

Incident
- with patient ☐
- with no patient ☐

Information
- education ☐
- prevention ☐
- agent ☐
- pharmaceutical ☐
- medico-legal ☐

Requested
- analyses ☐
- antidotes ☐
- printed material ☐
- identification ☐
- non-poisons information ☐

Others ☐

Unkown ☐

1.7 Status

☐ Emergency
☐ Non-emergency
☐ Unknown

1.8 Related to a previous Communication

☐ Yes
☐ No
☐ Unknown

1.8.1 Previous record

☐☐☐☐☐☐☐

1.9.1 Interlocutor (name)	Address	Phone
		Fax
1.9.2 Organization	Address	Phone
		Fax
1.9.3 Category*	1.9.4 Location*	

1.10 Custom ☐☐☐☐☐☐	1.11 Custom

1.12 Comments

_____
_____
_____
_____

2. INCIDENT		2.1 No ☐☐☐☐☐☐

2.2 Related to previous communication/incident	2.2.1 Communication no: ☐☐☐☐☐☐☐	2.2.2 Incident no: ☐☐☐☐☐☐☐

☐ Yes   ☐ No   ☐ Unknown

2.3 Type

Unintentional
- ☐ Accidental
- ☐ Occupational
- ☐ Environmental
- ☐ Transport/accident
- ☐ Fire
- ☐ Therapeutic error
- ☐ Misuse
- ☐ Food poisoning
- ☐ Other
- ☐ Unknown

Intentional
- ☐ Suicide
- ☐ Misuse
- ☐ Abuse
- ☐ Malicious/criminal
- ☐ Abortion
- ☐ Other
- ☐ Unknown

☐ Adverse reaction

☐ Other

☐ Unknown

2.4 Location*

2.5.1 Number of patients ☐☐☐☐	2.5.2 Group*

2.6 Custom ☐☐☐☐☐☐	2.7 Custom

2.8 Comments

_____
_____

INTOX-COMMUNICATION RECORD (continued)   Page 2 of 4
Version 3

3.1 No [ ][ ][ ][ ][ ][ ]

3. PATIENT

3.2 Type

☐ Human   ☐ Animal   ☐ Unknown

3.3 Species:*

3.4 Name:

Last name   First   Middle Initial

3.5 Hospital Record Number
[ ][ ][ ][ ][ ][ ][ ][ ][ ][ ][ ]

3.6 Address

3.7 Phone

3.8 Sex

☐ Male
☐ Female
☐ Unkown

3.9 Date of birth   dd   mm   yy
[ ][ ] [ ][ ] [ ][ ]

3.10 Age value

3.11 Age category

3.12 Ethnic origin*

3.13 Marital status

3.14.1 Pregnant

☐ Yes   ☐ Uncertain
☐ No   ☐ Unknown

3.14.2 Duration (weeks)
[ ][ ][ ]

3.15 Lactating?

☐ Yes   ☐ Unknown
☐ No

3.16 Height value

3.17 Weight value

3.18 Factors affecting susceptibility of the patient

3.18.1 Genetic _____

3.18.2 Previous medical history _____
_____
_____
_____

3.18.3 Other factors _____
_____
_____

3.19 Occupation

3.19.1 Patient*

3.19.2 Father/male guardian*

3.19.3 Mother/female guardian*

3.20 Clinical features
_____
_____
_____
_____

3.21 Symptoms/signs related to exposure

☐ Yes
☐ No
☐ Unknown
☐ Some

3.22 Initial severity grading

☐ None
☐ Minor
☐ Moderate
☐ Severe

3.23 Custom
[ ][ ][ ][ ][ ]

3.24 Custom

3.25 Comments
_____
_____
_____
_____

INTOX-COMMUNICATION RECORD (continued)   Page 3 of 4
Version 3

3. PATIENT (continued)

3.26 Management (*Put a check mark where applicable)

Treatment	3.26.1.1 Pre-enquiry	3.26.4.1 Recommended	3.26.5.1 Given
None			
Refused			
Oral Fluids			
Demulcents			
Neutralizing agent			
Gastric lavage			
Induced emesis -- ipecac			
Induced emesis -- other			
Activated charcoal (single dose)			
Activated charcoal (double dose)			
Cathartics			
Whole bowel irrigation			
Endoscopic removal			
Skin decontamination			
Irrigation of eyes			
Symptomatic treatment			
Clinical observation			
Supportive treatment			
Resuscitation			
Modified diuresis			
Haemodialysis			
Peritoneal dialysis			
Exchange transfusion			
Haemoperfusion			
Surgical intervention			
Antidotes			
Other			
Unknown			

Location of Treatment (*Put a check mark where applicable)

Location of Treatment	3.26.1.3 Pre-enquiry	3.26.4.3 Recommended	3.26.5.3 Given
Location of poisoning -- non health care staff			
Location of poisoning -- health care staff			
During transportation -- non health care staff			
During transportation -- health care staff			
Other location -- non health care staff			
Other location -- health care staff			
Health centre -- health staff, not physician			
Health centre -- physician			
Hospital attendance (ER)			
Hospital admission			
Specialized unit			
Other			
Unknown			

Antidote

3.26.1.2 Before enquiry

3.26.4.2 Recommended

3.26.5.2 Given

3.26.2 Risk assessment

- [ ] No risk
- [ ] Minimal or low risk
- [ ] Risk not excluded
- [ ] Serious risk or established poisoning

3.26.3 Investigations requested

3.26.6 Duration of hospitalization

3.26.7 Final severity grading

- [ ] None
- [ ] Minor
- [ ] Moderate
- [ ] Severe

3.26.9 Outcome

- [ ] Full recovery
- [ ] Full but delayed recovery
- [ ] Unknown
- [ ] Sequelae
- [ ] Death

3.27 Custom

[ ][ ][ ][ ][ ][ ]

3.28 Custom

3.29 Comments

INTOX-COMMUNICATION RECORD (continued)　Page 4 of 4
Version 3

4. AGENT

4.1 Agent name (interlocutor)	Agent – actual use
4.2 Agent name (centre)	4.2.1 Agent category*
4.3.1 Amount (interlocutor)	4.3.2 Amount (interlocutor)

4.3.2.1 Amount of major constituents

4.3.4 Qualitative estimate:

☐ Not significant ☐ Small ☐ Moderate ☐ Large ☐ Massive

4.4.1 Exposure type

☐ Acute – single
☐ Acute – repeated
☐ Chronic
☐ Acute on chronic
☐ Unknown

4.4.2 Exposure route

☐ Ingestion　　☐ Injection　which?.....
☐ Inhalation　☐ Mucosal　which?.....
☐ Cutaneous
☐ Otic/aural
☐ Ocular
☐ Bite
☐ Sting
☐ Placental
☐ Other
☐ Unknown

4.4.3 Time since last exposure	4.4.5.2 Units	4.4.5.3 Validity*
☐☐☐☐	☐ Seconds ☐ Days ☐ Months ☐ Minutes ☐ Weeks ☐ Years ☐ Hours	

4.4.4 If applicable, duration of single exposure 4.4.4.1 Value ☐☐☐☐	4.4.4.2 Units ☐ Seconds ☐ Days ☐ Months ☐ Minutes ☐ Weeks ☐ Years ☐ Hours	4.4.4.3 Validity*

4.4.5 Frequency and duration of multiple exposures

4.5 Correctness of information

4.6 Custom	4.7 Custom
☐☐☐☐☐☐	

4.8 Comments

Miniform

ID Number: Date: Time:

Interlocutor name: Phone:

Category: ▾   Location: ▾

Type of incident: ▾   Location: ▾

Patient name:

Patient age: ▾   Weight: ○ Male   ○ Female   ☐ Pregnant

Interlocutor agent: [Centre agent]

Agent quantity: ▾   Route of exposure: Time since last exposure:

Exposure type: ▾   ▾   ▾

Risk assessment: ▾   Duration of exposure: ▾

Initial severity: ▾

Final severity: ▾   [Clinical features]

Outcome: ▾   [Actual use]

Treatment before: ▾   [Investigation]

Treat. recommended: ▾   [Comments]

Treatment given: ▾

Annex 6

Proposed format for a poison centre annual report[1]

Period covered by the report: from .. / .. / .... to .. / .. / ....
                                  D M Y   D M Y

1. **Centre**

   Name:

   Address:

   Telephone:

   Fax:

   E-mail:

   Geographical area (officially) covered by centre:

   Population served (officially) by centre (*number*):

   Time of coverage: .... hours/day, from ..:.. to ..:.. .... days/week

   User profile:
   General public
   Medical professionals

   Type of service of centre:
   Poison information service
   Analytical
   Patient care
   Training
   Other

   Staff:
   Name of Technical/Medical Director:
   Name of Administrative Director:
   Professional: (*number*) (*indicate whether full-time or part-time*)
   Physicians
   Pharmacists
   Nurses
   Laboratory staff
   Other

   Administrative (*number*):

   General service (*number*):

   External experts/advisers (*number*):

---

[1] This is a suggested and somewhat comprehensive outline, which centres may wish to adapt for their own situation. Work is in progress in IPCS to establish an internationally agreed format with harmonized definitions of terms used in each section, following those used in the IPCS INTOX Package.

Fields of expertise (*e.g. agronomy, environment, botany, entomology*):

Date centre established (*date when service started operating*): .. / .. / ....

$\qquad\qquad\qquad\qquad\qquad\qquad\qquad\qquad\qquad$ D M Y

Location of centre (*e.g. ministry, hospital, medical school, university, other*):

Administrative affiliation (*e.g. Ministry of Health, university hospital, private sector, other*):

2. **Statistical data on communications**[1]

(a) Number of incoming, outgoing and other communications during reporting period (*communications by telephone, fax/telex, letter, personal contacts*), for example:

Telephone call		Letter		Fax/Telex		Questionnaire		Personal contacts	Other
In	Out	In	Out	In	Out	In	Out		

(b) Number of incoming communications including "personal contacts" that are requests for information only (NB: no exposure and no patient involved; all items that start with "Request for .....")

(c) Number of incoming communications including "personal contacts" concerning incidents only (NB: no patient involved)

(d) Number of incoming communications including "personal contacts" concerning incidents with patients

(e) Number of incoming communications per category of interlocutor (all)

(f) Number of incoming communications by location of interlocutor (all)

(g) Number of incoming communications including "personal contacts" per main category of use of agent

(h) Number of incoming communications including "personal contacts" by class of agent

(i) Number of incoming communications by month (*graphic presentation*):

(j) Number of incoming communications by hour of the day (yearly average) (*graphic presentation*)

(k) Comments

3. **Statistical data on incidents reported**[2]

(a) Total number of incidents reported

(b) Number of incidents involving more than one patient

(c) Number of incidents by type (*intentional, unintentional, adverse reaction, other, unknown*)

---

[1] A "communication" is any interaction between a centre and its interlocutors or clients.
[2] An incident relates to an event or episode in which an exposure or poisoning may or may not have taken place.

(d) Number of incidents by location (all)

(e) Number of incidents per main category of plant, fungus, or animal, or of agent (by use).

(f) Number of incidents per class of agent (*e.g. pharmaceutical; veterinary product; industrial/commercial product; household/leisure product; cosmetic/personal hygiene product; pesticide; agricultural product; abuse; food/beverage; warfare/anti-riot agent; environmental contaminant; other*)

(g) Comments

4. **Statistical data on patients involved in communications**[1]

(a) Total number of patients about whom communications are received
   — human (NB: this number should be the same as 2(d))
   — animal[2]

(b) Number of human patients by type of incident and agents by main category of use, e.g.

	Intentional	Unintentional	Adverse reaction	Other	Unknown	Total
Pharmaceuticals						
Veterinary products						
Industrial/commercial chemicals						
Household/leisure products						
Cosmetics/personal hygiene products						
Pesticides						
Agrochemicals, other than pesticides						
Abuse						
Food and beverages						
Warfare/anti-riot agents						
Environmental contaminants						
Other/unknown						
Total						

(c) Number of human patients by type of incident and by class of agent

(d) Number of human patients by type of incident and age groups and sex of patients

(e) Number of pregnant human patients

---

[1] This refers to data on humans or animals that have been exposed to or poisoned by an agent.
[2] Animal information given here.

(f) Number of human patients by age group and main category of use of the agent

(g) Number of human patients by age group and class of agent (NB: second or other level of the existing classification)

(h) Number of human patients by risk assessment

(i) Number of human patients by final severity grading

(j) Number of human patients by final outcome

(k) Number of human patients by treatment recommended by centre

(l) Number of human patients by location of treatment given before the enquiry

(m) Number of human patients by age group where outcome is death and type of incident

(n) Number of human patients by sex where outcome is death and main category of use of agent

(o) Number of human patients by sex where outcome is death and class of agent

(p) Comments (*e.g. summary of main observations, trends, general problems in relation to each main category of agent and specific problems with each category, such as cases with unusual symptomatology*)

5. Data on analytical and other laboratory investigations

(a) Type and quantity of analytical equipment operational in the laboratory[1]

(b) Total number of toxicological analytical investigations undertaken

(c) Total number of other laboratory investigations undertaken

(d) Main agents investigated and techniques used, in decreasing order of frequency

(e) Other investigations carried out by the laboratory:
   — identification of poisonous plants
   — identification of poisonous or venomous animal
   — analysis of water for chemical pollutants
   — analysis of food for chemical pollutants
   — analysis of food/water for microbiological pollutants
   — identification of controlled/abused drugs (seizures)
   — urine screening of drug abusers
   — forensic toxicology
   — occupational toxicology
   — environmental toxicology
   — therapeutic drug monitoring
   — clinical microbiology
   — others (*specify*)

(f) Comments (*e.g. availability of supplies and reagents*)

---

[1] For list of equipment and techniques for the analytical toxicology laboratory, see pages 39 and 42.

6. **Data on facilities for the management of patients**

(a) List number of beds (*e.g. in the centre itself, emergency room, intensive care unit, medical ward, other*)

(b) Outpatient clinic (*e.g. number of consultations*)

(c) Access to specialized treatment (*e.g. haemodialysis*)

(d) Access to specialized diagnostic facilities (*e.g. nuclear magnetic resonance*)

(e) Comments

7. **Antidotes and antivenoms available at centre**

(a) Antidotes and antivenoms available, used and distributed during the year[1]

(b) Comments (*e.g. new formulations and developments*)

8. **Prevention activities**

(a) Community poisoning prevention activities, including material prepared (*e.g. mass media activities, public education campaigns, other*)

(b) Partners in prevention activities (*e.g. ministries, hospitals, community groups, nongovernmental organizations, other*)

(c) Toxicovigilance activities:
    — number of investigations of toxic situations thought to require alert
    — number of alerts called
    — summary of reports to authorities and other actions taken
    — material prepared

(d) Results/outcome of prevention activities

(e) Comments

9. **Advisory roles to governmental and other bodies**

    (*e.g. Advice given on registration of pesticides, on safety measures, regulatory activities, other*)

10. **Training and education activities for professionals**

(a) Training courses organized by centre (*e.g. title, objectives, place, dates, type of audience, sponsorship, other*)

(b) Training activities organized by others where members of the centre took an active part (*e.g. title, objective, place, dates, type of audience, sponsorship, other*)

(c) Curricular studies organized by centre:
    — undergraduate level
    — postgraduate level

(d) Comments

11. **Research activities of the centre**

    (*e.g. titles, objectives, partners, duration, source of funding specifically for research, other*)

---

[1] For classified list of antidotes, see Annex 2.

(a) Clinical

(b) Analytical

(c) Epidemiological

(d) Projects

(e) Other

(f) Comments

12. **Publications**

(a) Publications/reports/brochures issued by the centre (*e.g. title, brief summary, reference*)

(b) Publications (*e.g. case reports, articles, monographs, theses, books*) written by the staff of the centre (*title, brief summary, and reference*)

(c) Comments

13. **Informatics facilities at centre**

(a) Computer hardware
    — type and number of computers
    — number of printers, CD-ROM drivers, tape drivers

(b) Computer software:
    — commercially available software (name and uses)
    — custom-built software (name and uses)

(c) Comments

14. **National and international meetings and cooperative activities of centre**

(a) Organized by the centre
    — national meetings/congresses/workshops (*e.g. title, place, dates, whether summary of meeting is available, number of members of the centre involved*)
    — international meetings/congresses/workshops (*e.g. title, place, dates, whether summary of meeting is available, number of members of the centre involved*)

(b) Participation of the centre
    — in national meetings/congresses/workshops (*e.g. title, place, dates, whether summary of meeting is available, number of members of the centre involved*)
    — in international meetings/congresses/workshops (*e.g. title, place, dates, whether summary of meeting is available, number of members of the centre involved*)

(c) Cooperative projects/activities (*e.g. title, brief description, partners, duration*)

(d) Support to other centres (e.g. setting up) (*brief description of activities, centre supported, dates, staff of the centre involved*)

(e) Training activities for other centres (*brief description, centre, dates*)

(f) Regional activities (*free-text description of activities in chronological order*)

(g) Comments

15. **Budget for the period of the report**

    (*local currency = US$ = other*)

(a) Overall annual budget

(b) Staff costs

(c) Operating costs

(d) Overall increase/decrease on previous year's budget

(e) Fund allocations for specific new activities (*e.g. activity, duration, amount*)

16. **Library resources at centre**

(a) Number of subscriptions (*list to be produced only for the first annual report*)

(b) List of new acquisitions in reporting period

(c) Comments

17. **Main needs of the centre**

This section is intended to present briefly the needs the centre has identified where technical, financial, or other support would be desirable, or where interaction with other centres would be fruitful.

Annex 7
The Environmental Health Criteria Series

The Environmental Health Criteria Series is published by WHO and may be obtained from Distribution and Sales, World Health Organization, 1211 Geneva 27, Switzerland.

Acetaldehyde (No. 167, 1995)
Acetonitrile (No. 154, 1993)
Acrolein (No. 127, 1991)
Acrylamide (No. 49, 1985)
Acrylonitrile (No. 28, 1983)
Aged population, principles for evaluating the effects of chemicals on (No. 144, 1992)
Aldicarb (No. 121, 1991)
Aldrin and dieldrin (No. 91, 1989)
Allethrins (No. 87, 1989)
Aluminium (in preparation)
Aluminosilicates (bentonite, etc.) (in preparation)
Amitrole (No. 158, 1994)
Ammonia (No. 54, 1986)
Anticoagulant rodenticides (No. 175, 1995)
Arsenic (No. 18, 1981)
Asbestos and other natural mineral fibres (No. 53, 1986)
Barium (No. 107, 1990)
Benomyl (No. 148, 1993)
Benzene (No. 150, 1993)
Beryllium (No. 106, 1990)
Biomarkers and risk assessment: concepts and principles (No. 155, 1993)
Biotoxins, aquatic (marine and freshwater) (No. 37, 1984)
Brominated diphenylethers (No. 162, 1994)
Butanols — four isomers (No. 65, 1987)
Cadmium (No. 134, 1992)
Cadmium — environmental aspects (No. 135, 1992)
Camphechlor (No. 45, 1984)
Carbamate pesticides: a general introduction (No. 64, 1986)
Carbaryl (No. 153, 1994)
Carbendazim (No. 149, 1993)
Carbon disulfide (No. 10, 1979)
Carbon monoxide (No. 13, 1979)
Carcinogens, summary report on the evaluation of short-term *in vitro* tests (No. 47, 1985)
Carcinogens, summary report on the evaluation of short-term *in vivo* tests (No. 109, 1990)
Chemical exposures, principles for assessment of risks from (Part A) (in preparation)
Chlordane (No. 34, 1984)

Chlordecone (No. 43, 1984)

Chlorendic acid and anhydride (No. 185, 1996)

Chlorinated flame retardants (in preparation)

Chlorinated paraffins (No. 181, 1996)

Chlorine and hydrogen chloride (No. 21, 1982)

Chlorobenzenes other than hexachlorobenzene (No. 128, 1991)

Chlorofluorocarbons, fully halogenated (No. 113, 1990)

Chlorofluorocarbons, partially halogenated

  (ethane derivatives) (No. 139, 1992)

  (methane derivatives) (No. 126, 1991)

Chloroform (No. 163, 1994)

Chlorophenols (No. 93, 1989)

Chlorothalonil (No. 183, 1996)

Chromium (No. 61, 1988)

Community noise (in preparation)

Cresols (No. 168, 1995)

Cyhalothrin (No. 99, 1990)

Cypermethrin (No. 82, 1989)

Cypermethrin, alpha- (No. 142, 1992)

DDT and its derivatives (No. 9, 1979)

DDT and its derivatives — environmental aspects (No. 83, 1989)

Deltamethrin (No. 97, 1990)

Diaminotoluenes (No. 74, 1987)

1,2-Dibromoethane (No. 177, 1996)

1,2-Dichloroethane (No. 62, 1987) (No. 176, 1995, 2nd ed.)

2,4-Dichlorophenoxyacetic acid (2,4-D) (No. 29, 1984)

2,4-Dichlorophenoxyacetic acid — environmental aspects (No. 84, 1989)

1,3-Dichloropropene, 1,2-dichloropropane and mixtures (No. 146, 1993)

Dichlorvos (No. 79, 1988)

Diesel fuel and exhaust emissions (No. 171, 1996)

Diethylhexyl phthalate (No. 131, 1992)

Diflubenzuron (No. 184, 1996)

Dimethoate (No. 90, 1989)

Dimethylformamide (No. 114, 1991)

Dimethyl sulfate (No. 48, 1985)

Diseases of suspected chemical etiology and their prevention, principles of studies on

  (No. 72, 1987)

Dithiocarbamate pesticides, ethylenethiourea, and propylenethiourea: a general intro-

  duction (No. 78, 1988)

Electromagnetic fields (No. 137, 1992)

Endosulfan (No. 40, 1984)

Endrin (No. 130, 1992)

Environmental epidemiology, guidelines on studies in (No. 27, 1983)

Epichlorohydrin (No. 33, 1984)

Ethylbenzene (No. 186, 1996)

Ethylene dibromide (in preparation)

Ethylene oxide (No. 55, 1985)

Extremely low frequency (ELF) fields (No. 35, 1984)

Fenitrothion (No. 133, 1992)

Fenvalerate (No. 95, 1990)

Fluorines and fluorides (No. 36, 1984)

Food additives and contaminants in food, principles for the safety assessment of (No. 70, 1987)

Formaldehyde (No. 89, 1989)

Genetic effects in human populations, guidelines for the study of (No. 46, 1985)

Glyphosate (No. 159, 1994)

Guidance values for health-based exposure limits (No. 170, 1994)

Heptachlor (No. 38, 1984)

Hexachlorobutadiene (No. 156, 1994)

Hexachlorocyclohexanes, alpha- and beta- (No. 123, 1992)

Hexachlorocyclopentadiene (No. 120, 1991)

n-Hexane (No. 122, 1991)

Hydrazine (No. 68, 1987)

Hydrogen sulfide (No. 19, 1981)

Hydroquinone (No. 157, 1994)

Immunotoxicity associated with exposure to chemicals: principles and methods for assessment (No. 180, 1996)

Infancy and early childhood, principles for evaluating health risks from chemicals during (No. 59, 1986)

Inorganic lead (No. 165, 1995)

Isobenzan (No. 129, 1991)

Isophorone (No. 174, 1995)

Kelevan (No. 66, 1986)

Lasers and optical radiation (No. 23, 1982)

Lead (No. 3, 1977)[1]

Lead — environmental aspects (No. 85, 1989)

Lead, inorganic (No. 165, 1995)

Lindane (No. 124, 1991)

Linear alkylbenzene sulfonates and selected related compounds (No. 169, 1995)

Magnetic fields (No. 69, 1987)

Man-made mineral fibres (No. 77, 1988)

Manganese (No. 17, 1981)

Mercury (No. 1, 1976)[1]

Mercury — environmental aspects (No. 86, 1989)

Mercury, inorganic (No. 118, 1991)

Methomyl (No. 178, 1996)

2-Methoxyethanol, 2-ethoxyethanol, and their acetates (No. 115, 1990)

Methyl bromide (No. 166, 1995)

Methylene chloride (No. 32, 1984, 1st ed.) (No. 164, 1996, 2nd ed.)

Methyl ethyl ketone (No. 143, 1992)

Methyl isobutyl ketone (No. 117, 1992)

Methyl isocyanate (in preparation)

Methylmercury (No. 101, 1990)

Methyl parathion (No. 145, 1992)

Mirex (No. 44, 1984)

Morpholine (No. 179, 1996)

Mutagenic and carcinogenic chemicals, guide to short-term tests for detecting (No. 51, 1985)

Mycotoxins (No. 11, 1979)

Mycotoxins, selected: ochratoxins, trichothecenes, ergot (No. 105, 1990)

Nephrotoxicity associated with exposure to chemicals, principles and methods for the assessment of (No. 119, 1991)

Neurotoxicity associated with exposure to chemicals, principles and methods for the
   assessment of (No. 60, 1986)

Nickel (No. 108, 1991)

Nitrates, nitrites, and N-nitroso compounds (No. 5, 1978)[1]

Nitrogen, oxides of (NO$_x$) (No. 4, 1977)[1] (No. 188, 1997, 2nd ed.)

2-Nitropropane (No. 138, 1992)

Noise (No. 12, 1980)[1]

Organophosphorus flame retardants (in preparation)

Organophosphorus insecticides: a general introduction (No. 63, 1986)

Paraquat and diquat (No. 39, 1984)

Pentachlorophenol (No. 71, 1987)

Permethrin (No. 94, 1990)

Pesticide residues in food, principles for the toxicological assessment of (No. 104, 1990)

Petroleum products, selected (No. 20, 1982)

Phenol (No. 161, 1994)

d-Phenothrin (No. 96, 1990)

Phosgene (in preparation)

Phosphine and selected metal phosphides (No. 73, 1988)

Photochemical oxidants (No. 7, 1978)

Platinum (No. 125, 1991)

Polybrominated biphenyls (No. 152, 1994)

Polychlorinated biphenyls and terphenyls (No. 2, 1976)[1] (No. 140, 1992, 2nd ed.)

Polychlorinated dibenzo-p-dioxins and dibenzofurans (No. 88, 1989)

Progeny, principles for evaluating health risks associated with exposure to chemicals
   during pregnancy (No. 30, 1984)

1-Propanol (No. 102, 1990)

2-Propanol (No. 103, 1990)

Propachlor (No. 147, 1993)

Propylene oxide (No. 56, 1985)

Pyrrolizidine alkaloids (No. 80, 1988)

Quintozene (No. 41, 1984)

Quality management for chemical safety testing (No. 141, 1992)

Radiofrequency and microwaves (No. 16, 1981)

Radionuclides, selected (No. 25, 1983)

Resmethrins (No. 92, 1989)

Selenium (No. 58, 1986)

Styrene (No. 26, 1983)

Sulfur oxides and suspended particulate matter (No. 8, 1979)

Synthetic organic fibres, selected (No. 151, 1993)

Tecnazene (No. 42, 1984)

Tetrabromobisphenol A and derivatives (No. 172, 1995)

Tetrachloroethylene (No. 31, 1984)

Tetradifon (No. 67, 1986)

Tetramethrin (No. 98, 1990)

Thallium (No. 182, 1996)

Thiocarbamate pesticides: a general introduction (No. 76, 1988)

Tin and organotin compounds (No. 15, 1980)

Titanium (No. 24, 1982)

Toluene (No. 52, 1986)

---

[1] Out of print.

Toluene diisocyanates (No. 75, 1987)
Toxicity of chemicals (Part 1), principles and methods for evaluating (No. 6, 1978)
Toxicokinetic studies, principles of (No. 57, 1986)
Tributyl phosphate (No. 112, 1991)
Tributyltin compounds (No. 116, 1990)
Trichlorfon (No. 132, 1992)
1,1,1-Trichloroethane (No. 136, 1992)
Trichloroethylene (No. 50, 1985)
Tricresyl phosphate (No. 110, 1990)
Triphenyl phosphate (No. 111, 1991)
Tris- and bis(2,3-dibromophenyl) phosphate (No. 173, 1995)
Ultrasound (No. 22, 1982)
Ultraviolet radiation (No. 14, 1979) (No. 160, 1994, 2nd ed.)
Vanadium (No. 81, 1988)
Vinylidene chloride (No. 100, 1990)
White spirit (No. 187, 1996)
Xylenes (No. 190, 1997)

Selected WHO publications of related interest

Basic analytical toxicology
Flanagan RJ et al.
1995 (xii + 274 pages + 8 colour plates)
Sw. fr. 60.–

Management of poisoning. A handbook for health care personnel
Henry J, Wiseman H (in press)

Safe use of pesticides
Fourteenth Report of the WHO Expert Committee
on Vector Biology and Control
WHO Technical Report Series, No. 813, 1991 (iv + 27 pages)
Sw. fr. 6.–

Public health impact of pesticides used in agriculture
1990 (128 pages)
Sw. fr. 21.–

Trace elements in human nutrition and health
1996 (xviii + 343 pages)
Sw. fr. 85.–

Laboratory biosafety manual, 2nd ed.
1993 (144 pages)
Sw. fr. 26.–

Screening and surveillance of workers exposed to mineral dusts
Wagner GR
1997 (ix + 68 pages)
Sw. fr. 24.–

Our planet, our health
Report of the WHO Commission on Health and Environment
1992 (xxxii + 282 pages)
Sw. fr. 45.–

Further information on these and other WHO publications can be obtained from
Distribution and Sales, World Health Organization, 1211 Geneva 27, Switzerland.

Prices subject to change. Prices in developing countries are reduced by 30%.